Ayurveda and Marma Therapy

Energy Points
in Yogic Healing

By Dr. David Frawley,
Dr. Subhash Ranade
and Dr. Avinash Lele

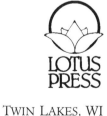

LOTUS
PRESS

TWIN LAKES, WI

Cover & Page Design/Layout: Paul Bond, Art & Soul Design
Illustrations: Vijay Bagore

First Edition, 2003

Second Printing, 2005

Third Printing, 2008

Printed in the United States of America

Ayurveda and Marma Therapy: Energy Points in Yogic Healing includes bibliographical references.

ISBN: 978-0-9409-8559-9

Library of Congress Control Number: 2003102519

Published by:
Lotus Press, P.O. Box 325, Twin Lakes, Wisconsin 53181
web: www.lotuspress.com
e-mail: lotuspress@lotuspress.com
800-824-6396

Table of Contents

We would like to thank various people
for helping us with the book.

For the Illustrations:
Vijay Bagore who did the main illustrations of the marma points.
Swami Sada Shiva Tirtha of *The Ayurveda Encyclopedia*
for help with the black and white drawings.

Those who have given important
comments and suggestions to the text:
Alan Christianson, Atreya Smith, Sandra Kozak.

Proofing and copyediting:
Betheyla Anuradha

Dr. Frank Ros for his chapter on Marmapuncture

Foreword

The subject of pranic energy as a biological force is well documented in Ayurveda, but until now, poorly understood in the West. Prana as the positive energy of the *vata dosha* is the primary source of physical and energetic health. Ayurvedic medicine has a wonderful therapeutic system to work directly on this bio-energetic principle that is called Marma therapy.

Prana as the source of the *tridosha* is the single most important factor in health and therapeutic treatment. All Ayurvedic therapies work on the prana of the patient in some manner, striving to stabilize and harmonize its functions, primarily through the three doshas, *vata*, *pitta* and *kapha*. Marma therapy is the most direct method of harmonizing prana in the physical body (*Sthula sharira*) of another person. It can also aid in the study of yoga practices such as pranayama and asana, which are chiefly concerned with increasing and regulating pranic function through the *nadis* or channels of the subtle body. Marma therapy supplements and supports all Ayurvedic therapies, increasing their effectiveness and ability to awaken the healing power of the body.

Prana as the source of mental function and perception allows us to think and perceive. It allows us to interact with the five senses, body and physical universe. The higher forms of Yoga are concerned with the development of prana on this level, the subtle body (*Sukshma sharira*), which governs the mind and senses. The advanced aspects of Ayurveda can assist to harmonize prana here and aid in all forms of personal development and spiritual unfoldment. Marma therapy plays a key role in bridging the physical and subtle bodies of yogic science. Therefore, a working knowledge of Marma therapy is an important assistance on all yogic paths. Thus, Marma therapy is a multidimensional approach to health that includes the physical, energetic and mental sheaths (*Annamaya*, *Pranamaya* and *Manomaya Koshas*) that in turn have an effect on the souls apparent journey home.

Marma therapy is used as a part of most Ayurvedic treatments and is of primary importance in self-care and self-healing. Indian doctors prescribe it as a matter of course for patients who are also taking herbal or other Ayurvedic medicines. Yet, Marma therapy is used alone to treat a variety of disorders ranging from paralyses to psychosomatic disorders. The uses of Marma therapy are almost unlimited for health care and form a corner stone of classical Ayurvedic medicine.

For the first time we are presented with a clear book on the subject from three world famous authors, lecturers and doctors. *Ayurveda and Marma Therapy* is an updated and revised edition first published in India. The present edition goes far beyond the old and adds much practical information for the Western therapist of massage and acupressure. A number of misconceptions and confusions are cleared up in this edition to form a clear, practical therapeutic guide for the Westerner. In short, the present edition of this landmark work has little to do with the original and is much improved.

The main confusion regarding Marma therapy in the West is the concept of 107 fixed points on the physical anatomy. In reality the Ayurvedic vision of marma points is flexible and adapted to the individual, as are all Ayurvedic therapies. The marma points can differ from one individual to another and require a certain sensitivity on the part of the therapist to find the area of pranic congestion. In practice we find a variety of differences manifesting according to the *prakriti* (constitution) and *vikriti* (temporary state) of the person. Applying the information in this book too rigidly would be a disservice and would ignore the main vision of Ayurveda as an individualized medicine.

There are also a number of minor marma points that are not classified under the primary 107 points. Additionally, the ancient restriction on the use of Marma therapy by unqualified persons shows the need of respect and sensitivity when working on these dynamic points of energy. Furthermore, there are regional differences on marma location in India. What we may learn in Western India can be different from Northern or Southern India. There are also different approaches from different doctors or practitioners. While this may seem confusing to the beginner it actually adds to the richness of the tradition and forces the practitioner to use his or her intelligence when applying the marma system to a patient. After all, the main purpose of Ayurveda is for us to become more intelligent. *Ayurveda and Marma Therapy* assists everyone in this endeavor with clear, profound knowledge.

Atreya Smith

Author of *Secrets of Ayurvedic Massage*; *Perfect Balance, Ayurvedic Nutrition*; and director of the European Institute of Vedic Studies in France.

Preface

The science of Yoga, which has become very popular all over the world in recent decades, is intimately connected to Ayurveda as its corresponding system of natural medicine. As Yoga and Ayurveda become better known, more interest is developing in their specific healing modalities as well. A new Yoga and Ayurveda therapy is arising, integrating their renewed mutual application using yogic tools like asana according to Ayurvedic guidelines as well as applying Ayurvedic therapies to aid in yogic healing.

The use of pressure points, called marmas in Sanskrit, is an important part of this Yoga/Ayurveda interface. Marmas are a common topic in classical Ayurvedic texts and are referred to in modern books as well. They are also frequently mentioned in yogic teachings. But up to this present volume— *Ayurveda and Marma Therapy* —there is no single book that attempts to make this subject easily accessible and readable in the West. This book is meant to help fill in that gap.

Ayurveda and Marma Therapy has three authors: Dr. David Frawley (Pandit Vamadeva Shastri) of the USA along with Dr. Subhash Ranade and Dr. Avinash Lele both of Pune, India. Dr. Frawley is one of the leading western Ayurvedic experts, having authored half a dozen books on the subject as well as developed extensive course material for Ayurvedic programs. He has taken the main lead in shaping the book. Dr. Ranade is one of the most important Indian Ayurvedic doctors teaching in the western world as well as in India. He has written many books, including textbooks used in Ayurvedic colleges. Dr. Ranade and Dr. Frawley co-authored the book *Ayurveda: Nature's Medicine*. Dr. Lele, a colleague of Dr. Ranade, is another important Ayurvedic doctor who has specialized in marma therapy. He is trained in traditional Ayurvedic methods of surgery, which carefully considers the use of marmas. Dr. Ranade and Dr. Lele have collaborated on several Ayurvedic books published in India.

Dr. Frawley wrote the greater portion of the material in the book, including the explanations of Ayurvedic principles and treatments in the first section, as well as most of the information on the treatment of marmas in the Table of Marmas in the second section. He specifically developed the material explaining the use of marmas relative to the practice of Yoga and meditation, including their treatment with gem and color therapy, drawing on various yogic teachings and other related Vedic sciences. Dr. Ranade and Dr. Lele provided the illustrations and most of the information on the description of marma points, as well as the initial outline of the book.

The book aims both at identifying marmas and indicating the appropriate methods to treat them effectively. Such methods include massage with special oils, herbs and aromas as well as acupressure, acupuncture and various herbal remedies. While classical Ayurvedic herbs and massage oils are presented for those who have access to these, we have also offered commonly available herbs and oils so that any interested reader can begin to use marma therapy for self-care purposes. The treatment of marmas with aroma therapy, which is quick and easy to do, has been a major topic.

We would like to offer a special thanks to Dr. Frank Ros, author of *The Lost Secrets of Ayurvedic Acupuncture* for his chapter on 'Marmapuncture', explaining Ayurvedic acupuncture in detail. Dr. Ros is perhaps the western world's foremost expert on this important topic.

We would like to emphasize that this book is not meant to present the last word on the number of marmas, their location or their manner of treatment. The book emphasizes the main classical Ayurvedic marmas, which are 107 in number, but many other such sensitive points can also be used. While it introduces various methods of treating marmas, particularly oil massage and aroma therapy, such methods can be delineated in greater detail and adapted relative to various treatment strategies and a comprehensive Ayurvedic therapy. The book is a good place to start working with marmas, but still only an introduction to this profound topic. It should be supplemented by a further study of Ayurveda for its full application and integration with the entire range of Ayurvedic modalities.

We have not dealt a great deal with how Ayurvedic marma therapy interfaces with the many forms of bodywork and massage that are practiced today. That is another vast field for research which, hopefully, other therapists will take up in time. We have included several references in the bibliography for those who wish to take up related forms of Ayurvedic healing, energy healing or bodywork. We welcome any feedback from our readers, in order to improve any future editions of this book in light of their suggestions.

Ayurveda remains a vast ocean and we are still but getting acquainted with its waves and currents. May we gain the power to sail into its endless horizons and enter new universes of healing and self-transformation!

Dr. David Frawley, Dr. Subhash Ranade & Dr. Avinash Lele
May 2002

Part One

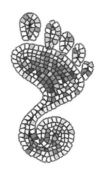

Introduction to Marmas: Energy Points of Yoga and Ayurveda

CHAPTER 1

Marmas: Energy Points of Yoga and Ayurveda

The use of pressure points for massage and acupuncture has become a popular topic in natural healing today. In Ayurveda, the traditional medicine of India, these pressure points are called *marmas*, meaning 'vulnerable' or 'sensitive' zones. Such points can be used specifically for the diagnosis and treatment of disease or generally for promoting health and longevity. Marmas are integral to all Ayurvedic therapies from simple self-treatments to complex clinical procedures. They form one of the main pillars of Ayurvedic thought and practice.

Marmas are also an important aspect of the science of Yoga, with which Ayurveda is closely connected. Yoga not only has a sophisticated system of physical postures, it also recognizes the power of Prana or the life-force, which is reflected through the marma points on the surface of the body. An understanding of marmas can add greater efficacy to any level or type of yoga practice whether using the body, the breath or the mind.

Just as acupuncture points are used in both Chinese medicine and in Chinese martial arts, marma points are also used in the martial arts of India, like the Kalari tradition of South India. Martial arts emphasize how to strike these vulnerable points with force and precision in order to counter attackers. The existence of such vital regions demonstrates that the body is not simply a physical mass but an intricate energy field with points of power through which we can control both physiological and psychological processes.

Marmas are part of a greater 'sacred physiology' that maps out the body according to subtle energy currents and power points. The body has its own special sacred points just as the Earth has its sacred sites and energy currents according to sacred geography. We must learn this sacred geography of our own body in order to attune ourselves both to the Earth and to the greater cosmos.

Without knowing these lines of force on our own bodies we cannot really understand ourselves or our interaction with our environment, nor can we create lasting balance and harmony in our lives. Yet though marmas are a key component to India's traditional sciences, not many people in the West know about them, including many who have studied Yoga or even Ayurveda. A study of marmas adds a new dimension of insight to both systems, helping us tap into the currents of vitality and creativity within and around us.

As a first step to understanding marmas, let us examine how they fit into the greater scheme of Yoga, Ayurveda and other Vedic sciences.

Ayurvedic Medicine and Marma Therapy

Ayurveda is India's traditional healing system, its profound system of mind-body medicine, natural living and yogic health. Ayurveda, which means 'the science of life', has become recognized today for its wonderful dietary, herbal, life-style and yogic therapies that help us live longer, happier, wiser and more in harmony with the greater universe of life and consciousness. Ayurveda was the dominant medical paradigm in the Indian subcontinent until modern times and is still widely practiced throughout the region as a complete medical system. Its roots go back deep both in time and in consciousness. Ayurveda is part of the older spiritual heritage of humanity that contains much secret knowledge and profound wisdom. It interfaces closely with the spiritual science of Yoga, and developed parallel to it both historically and in terms of its prime concepts.

The science of marma or *Marma Vidya* is another extraordinary and dynamic Ayurvedic therapy that has tremendous value in health, disease, everyday living and in spiritual practice. Marma therapy or *Marma Chikitsa* is an important method of Ayurvedic treatment for the entire spectrum of health complaints major and minor. Many different marma regions are described in Ayurvedic texts along with their specific effects on both body and mind. Marmas range in size from very small to very large, from special points along the hands and feet to significant regions on the trunk of the body like the heart or the navel. When manipulated, marmas can alter both the organic function and structural condition of the body. Through the right use of marmas our entire physical and mental energy can be consciously increased, decreased or redirected in a transformative manner.

Marmas resemble the acupuncture points of Traditional Chinese Medicine but extend to larger areas of the body. They include vital organs like the heart and bladder as well as bones and joints and points along the surface of the body. Marmas are centers for the vital-force or *Prana*, the master power behind both physical and psychological processes. Marmas serve like pranic switches that can be used to turn Prana up or down, on or off at various places on the body. Through manipulation of marmas, Prana can be directed to remove blockages, improve energy flow or tap hidden energy reserves and make connections with the greater powers of life and nature. This makes marma therapy an important tool of 'energetic' or 'pranic healing'.

The condition of marmas is an important diagnostic tool in Ayurveda. At marma sites toxins, stress and negative emotions get lodged and are held, sometimes for years. Disease is reflected in pain, blockage or swelling in these areas even before it may manifest outwardly in the full range of disease symptoms. Ayurvedic doctors palpate marmas as an integral part of patient examination and gain much information from them. Relieving pain, blockage or swelling at marma sites is an important therapeutic aid and one of the first stages of many Ayurvedic treatments.

Marmas are key locations for Ayurvedic bodywork and massage. The Ayurvedic massage therapist will focus on marma regions that are in need of stimulation or of release and use the appropriate methods to adjust their energy flow. Ayurveda treats marmas with pressure, heat, needles, massage oils, herbs or aromatic oils, providing many tools for working with our internal energies through them.

Marmas are a common topic in the three great Ayurveda classics of *Charaka, Sushruta* and *Vagbhatta*, which provide a wealth of information on their location, function and application. Marma therapy can be used along with all Ayurvedic therapies from detoxification to tonification and rejuvenation, from self-care to intricate clinical procedures like Pancha Karma.

Marmas and the System of Yoga

Marmas are key energy centers for the practice of yoga on all levels from yoga postures (Asanas) to deep meditation (Dhyana). Yoga postures affect the energy held in the limbs, joints and spine, which all contain important marmas. Asanas can be used to stimulate and balance marmas in various ways. Similarly, certain marmas can be manipulated while a person is performing various asanas in order to augment their effects.

Marmas connect to the *nadis* (subtle nerves) and *chakras* (energy centers) of the subtle body and the mind. They govern the interface between the physical and subtle (pranic) bodies and the interchange of energy and information between them. This means that marmas are important for healing the subtle body as well as the physical body. Through using marmas we can restore the proper connection between the subtle body (our internal energy, moods and emotions) and the physical body (our material condition), resulting in increased health and vitality on both levels.

As the important bodily sites in which Prana is located, marmas can be used along with yogic breathing practices (Pranayama). Through yogic breathing, we can direct Prana through different marmas for healing purposes, improving their energy flow from within. Marmas are key places where stress and attachment accumulate, blocking the free flow of energy and awareness. They can be treated through relaxation techniques and the yogic practice of *Pratyahara* (yogic internalization methods and sensory therapies) to release such blockages.

Marmas similarly have a place in higher Yoga practices of concentration, mantra and meditation. Special mantras can be used with particular marmas in order to increase physical or psychological strength, adaptability and immunity. Those who meditate regularly become sensitive to the condition of marmas and aware of the flow of energy through them, which they can learn to modify through thought and will power alone. Through developing mental concentration, meditators can learn to energize or clear marma points, without requiring any external aids.

Therefore, a good Yoga teacher should possess a good knowledge of marmas and how they relate to various Yoga practices. A serious Yoga student should not overlook the location or function of marmas in developing an effective practice.

Marmas and Vedic Sciences

The science of marma (Marma Vidya) is an integral part of all the 'Vedic' or 'yogic' sciences that emerged in India in ancient times. The *Rig Veda*, the oldest Vedic text, is a collection of *mantras*, which are words of power or primal sounds that mirror the workings of the universe on all levels. These Vedic mantras—the essence of which is the Divine word OM—reflect the 'cosmic marmas', the sensitive energy points that govern the greater universe and its processes. Just as mantras are the seed-powers that underlie speech and language, so marmas are the seed-sites that underlie the body and its movement.

The Vedic vision regards the entire universe or macrocosm as the cosmic person or *Purusha*, with the human body as a replica or miniature, a microcosm. This means that the mapping of the energy fields in the human body reflects that of the universe as a whole. The science of marma arose from this Vedic view that our Prana or life energy field adheres to the same pattern as the world of nature.

Originally marma was part of Vedic martial arts or *Dhanur Veda*, which is one of the four *Upavedas* or secondary *Vedas*.

Four Upavedas or Secondary Vedas

1. Dhanur Veda—Martial arts
2. Ayurveda—Medicine for both body and mind
3. Gandharva Veda—Music, dance and literature
4. Sthapatya Veda—Vastu or directional influences and architecture

Yet the science of marma is an important part of all Vedic sciences, connected to all Vedic disciplines from dance to astrology. It reflects the music of nature and the points at which our body can receive the influences of the four directions. It connects us to the cosmic rhythms through which our life reaches out to the universal life.

Marma, Tantra and Siddha Medicine

Marmas are particularly important in the Siddha system of medicine, a Tantric and South Indian form of Ayurveda. In the Siddha system, marmas are referred to under the term '*varma*', an old synonym for marma as a bodily site that requires protection. The Vedic rishi and sage *Agastya* is considered to be the founder of the science of varma.

According to the Siddha system, the entire universe originates from the union of Lord *Shiva*—Being (Sat)—and his wife *Parvati*—energy or consciousness-force (Cit-Shakti). Shiva is closely connected to Prana. Prana at rest is Shiva and in motion is Shakti. The use of marma or varma as a form of energy treatment connects to both Shiva and Shakti forces.

In Siddha thought, varma points are invisible but can be traced where body, mind and psychic energies concentrate together. As such, they are places where the vital energy in the body can become blocked.[1] This can be due either to external injuries or internal factors like fear or anger. Such blockages can be perceived as a kind of psychic energy. Therefore, marmas can be controlled by meditation, mantra, Pranayama and other yogic methods. Marmas can also be used for enhancing mental and spiritual powers. The Siddha system refers to marmas relative to the effects of the Moon and the planets on the human body, bringing in an astrological link as well.

Historical Background of Marmas

The science of marma can be traced along with the history of civilization and healing in ancient India, which is one of the oldest and most sophisticated civilizations in the world.[2] This begins with the ancient Indus-Sarasvati culture (3500-1700 BCE), the largest urban civilization of the world at that time, as revealed in large archaeological sites like Harappa, Mohenjodaro, Rakhigarhi and Dholavira,[3] most of which are located on the long dried-up Sarasvati River in North India.[4] The science of marma grew up along with other Vedic disciplines from this period, including the science of Yoga, which is evident from the many seals of figures in Yoga and meditation postures found in such sites. Early Vedic texts, probably dating from this time, describe major marma regions like the head, the heart and the navel, along with the various Pranas, and the tissues and organs of the body.[5]

After this long formative era came the classical period of Ayurveda (1700 BCE-700 AD) in which the main Ayurvedic texts were compiled like *Charaka Samhita, Sushruta Samhita, Ashtanga Hridaya* and *Ashtanga Sangraha*. These classics contain references to marmas, particularly Sushruta who was himself a surgeon. This was the same period in which yogic texts describing asana, Pranayama and nadis mentioned the use of marmas as well. In the later part of this period, the Buddhist religion spread Ayurveda, marma therapy and related martial arts east to China and Japan.

After this classical period came a long decline in Ayurveda, brought about by foreign invasions and colonial rule, which lasted up to modern times, in which many texts and practices were lost, including much significant information about marmas. Only during the recent period since India's independence in 1947 has a revival of Ayurveda brought about new research on topics like marma, which is now being viewed as one of the most important aspects of Ayurveda requiring a new critical examination and application.

Marmas and Martial Arts

The knowledge of marmas was part of the path of the warrior who learned to master his Prana for both defensive and offensive purposes. The ancient Vedic warrior code emphasized the development of personal energy, courage and self-discipline, which rested on the knowledge and control of Prana and its key sites within the body.

Marmas were associated with the use of armor for the body, called 'varma' in Sanskrit, which was devised to protect these vital points from injury. The first references to marma in the *Rig-Veda* speak of using varma or protective coverings to protect these marmas. It refers to prayer or mantra (Brahman) as the best protection (varma) for these marmas, showing a spiritual view behind the use of marmas from the very beginning. This tradition continued as the use of mantras for protective purposes.

The great epic *Mahabharata*, in which the *Bhagavad Gita* of Sri Krishna occurs, contains many references to marma and varma.[6] It mentions protective coverings for the marmas of elephants and horses as well of soldiers. At that time great warriors could use their powers of Prana and mental force (mantra) as fighting tools, energizing arrows with natural forces like fire or lightning. The *Mahabharata* details a number of such encounters between great warriors like Arjuna and Karna, who could only be defeated if their marma points were exposed.

Today these Vedic martial arts are best preserved in South India, where traditional martial arts like *Kalari Payat* (in Kerala) and *Kalari Payirchi* (in Tamil Nadu) are still commonly practiced. The highest form of martial arts is called Marma Adi or Varma Adi, in which the knowledge of marmas is central. From this art of self-defense originated the *Varma Kalai* or *Varma Chikitsa*, Marma or Varma therapy. Expert physicians in this therapy were highly regarded and often became royal physicians.[7]

The spiritual traditions of India have always emphasized the principle of *Ahimsa*— non-harming or non-violence as the basis of spiritual practices. Monks were not allowed to use weapons for self-defense, so martial arts were taught to them for unarmed self-protection. The Buddhist text *Milindapanha*, a dialogue between King Milinda and the monk Nagasena, dating from the second century BCE, explains unarmed self-defense as one of the nineteen monastic arts. Such martial arts gained prominence when Buddhism spread beyond the boundaries of India into China, Indonesia and Thailand, where the monks no longer had the protection of the kings that they generally had in India.

It is possible that Traditional Chinese Medicine adapted aspects of marma therapy, which has much in common with acupuncture, from Ayurveda and Siddha Medicine. Bodhidharma, who traditionally brought both Zen meditation and martial arts to China in the sixth century, is said to have originated from the famous South Indian town of Kanchipuram, a famous center of learning for yogic disciplines and one of the seven sacred cities of the subcontinent.

Yet whatever the history may be, marmas and similar energy practices have always been with us in one form or another and are an integral part of the new world medicine. They are experiencing a great revival again today in this age of new interest in natural healing and traditional spirituality.

---

[1] These points are called *maitheenda kala'*.

[2] Recent finds of an ancient city in the Gulf of Cambay (*India Today*, Feb. 2002) may go back well before 5000 BCE.

[3] Note books like *Gods, Sages and Kings* (Frawley) and *In Search of the Cradle of Civilization* (Feuerstein, Kak and Frawley).

[4] According to recent archaeology, the Sarasvati River dried up owing to geological changes, climate changes and the shifting of its headwaters, finishing the river as a perennial stream around 1900 BCE. Vedic culture must be older than that to know of this great river.

[5] Note the *Satapatha Brahmana* in this respect.

[6] For example, *Mahabharata Karnaparva* 19.31, *Shalyaparva* 32.63 and 36.64, *Dronaparva* 125.17, *Bhishmaparva* 95.47, *Virataparva* 31.12 and 15.

[7] In the Tamil language many manuscripts are available on this secret art like *Varma Soothiram, Varma Peerangi, Varma Thiravugole, Varma Ponosi, Varma Kundoci,* and *Varma Gurunadi*. These manuscripts describe in detail various types of marmas and their treatment.

CHAPTER 2

The Ayurvedic System of Healing and Marma Therapy

To properly approach marma therapy, we must understand its background in Ayurvedic medicine. The following chapter is a brief account of the Ayurvedic view of the body and the energies at work behind it, particularly relative to the use of marmas. The reader can consult additional books on Ayurveda for more details on this great system of natural medicine.[1]

Ayurveda like Yoga rests upon the ancient *Samkhya* system of cosmology for its theoretical background. The Samkhya system sets forth the 'worldview' of Yoga and Ayurveda, out of which their principles and practices evolved and which explains their goals. Samkhya recognizes two ultimate universal principles of spirit and matter, *Purusha* and *Prakriti*, or the 'consciousness' principle and the principle of 'form'. From the union of Purusha and Prakriti arises the entire universe on all levels from inanimate matter to living beings of all types.

Purusha is the 'pure consciousness' or 'higher Self' that is the ultimate source of life, awareness and feeling. The goal of human life is to realize this higher Self in which we can go beyond all suffering and pain, gaining release from karma and the cycle of birth and death. Connecting with the higher Self is the ultimate goal of Ayurvedic healing as well as that of Yoga practice.

Prakriti is Nature or the principle of manifestation in time and space, whose laws and processes underlie the body and mind and their interactions. Just as our consciousness or eternal nature is one with the higher Self, our body and mind or temporal manifestation follows the laws of Nature or Prakriti. In order to realize our higher Self and spiritual freedom (Purusha), we must first harmonize our embodiment (Prakriti). This means that balance and well-being in both body and mind are integral aspects of spiritual development and the foundation for deeper practices. We cannot ignore the body to find the spirit. Rather the body is our vehicle for realizing the spirit.

Relative to marmas as energy zones on the body, we could say that, on the highest level, marmas are places in the body where Purusha and Prakriti interface, where consciousness and Prana (Purusha) are reflected in our psycho-physical structure and dynamic (Prakriti). Marmas help us harmonize our Prakriti (our practical manifestation) and our Purusha (our quest for Self-realization).

The Three Gunas and the Five Elements

The Purusha is a homogenous entity composed of pure consciousness that serves as the seer and witness behind the processes of nature, which function through its presence. Prakriti or Nature, however, is a heterogeneous substance with diverse actions. It is composed of the three *gunas* or prime qualities of *sattva* (balance and intelligence) *rajas* (action and energy) and *tamas* (inertia or materiality) and their ever-changing permutations and interactions.

The gunas are the primordial forces behind cosmic evolution, which proceeds from matter (tamas) to life (rajas) and mind (sattva). Only from the level of pure sattva (the clarity of the higher mind) can we have an enduring access to the Purusha or higher Self, whose nature is extremely subtle. For this reason, both Yoga and Ayurveda emphasize the cultivation of sattva guna.[2] Marmas can be used to balance our Prana or vital energy and increase sattva.

From the combination of the three gunas arises the five great elements (Pancha Mahabhutas) of earth, water, fire, air and ether—the solid, liquid, radiant, gaseous and etheric forms of matter—which are central to both yogic and Ayurvedic thought. The elements show that the entire universe consists of different frequencies or vibrations of the same underlying substance (Prakriti), just as water can be found in solid, liquid and gaseous forms.

From these five great elements the three biological humors or *doshas* arise—the main factors of Ayurvedic thought. The doshas are the underlying energetic forces behind the workings of both body and mind. They represent the five elements imbued with the life-force (Prana). Each dosha consists of two of the five great elements as well as a portion of the three gunas.

ELEMENT	GUNA	DOSHA
Ether	Sattva	Vata
Air	Rajas	Vata
Fire	Sattva + Rajas	Pitta
Water	Sattva + Tamas	Kapha/Pitta
Earth	Tamas	Kapha

In this scheme, the subtle elements of air and ether (Vata dosha) control the gross elements of earth, water and fire (Kapha and Pitta doshas). Most marmas are located near joints and orifices that contain space and hold air or energy. Marmas are important centers that govern the air and ether elements in the body and therefore can be used to control the elements in the body as a whole.

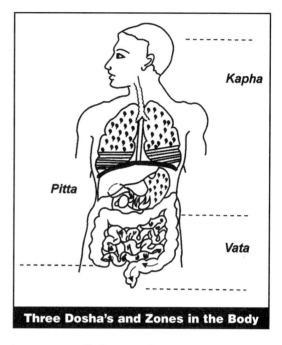

Three Dosha's and Zones in the Body

The Three Doshas

The three doshas or biological humors are the prime factors behind both health and disease. To understand them more easily, we can compare them to the three main forces at work in the atmosphere—with Vata as wind, Pitta as heat (particularly the force of the Sun), and Kapha as moisture (both on Earth and in the atmosphere). Wind, heat (temperature) and moisture in their interaction create all the weather patterns on Earth. They are responsible for all weather changes and the external climate as they fluctuate throughout the seasons.

Similarly, the three doshas rule over our internal climate or internal atmosphere by their ever changing interactions of movement (Vata), heat (Pitta) and moisture (Kapha) through the rhythms of time and the aging process. Health consists of the timely development and harmonious interaction of the three doshas. Disease is caused by their imbalances, excesses and inappropriate movements.

1. Vata Dosha
The Principle of Movement or Propulsion

- Vata means 'that which moves or conveys things'. It is composed of the ether and air elements, which are its conditions of rest (ether) and movement (air).
- Vata is responsible for all major and minor, perceptible and imperceptible movements in the body. It is the prime force that governs the transportation of fluids, the discharge of secretions, and the elimination of waste-materials. Its main physical disorders are tissue depletion,

debility, dehydration and disturbances to the mind and nervous system.

- Vata governs the mind and the senses, which function through its bio-electrical force, ensuring their quick and balanced function. It gives agility, adaptability and good communication skills to the mind. Emotionally, Vata's main disturbances are fear and anxiety. It causes ungroundedness and instability when imbalanced or when in excess.

- Vata's subtle or master form is *Prana* or the life-force, the prime vital energy behind all that we do. Prana is responsible for our organic equilibrium, hormonal secretions, growth, healing, creativity and rejuvenation. It is the master force behind all our states and conditions of body and mind.

- Vata's main site in the digestive system is the *large intestine* where it accumulates in the form of waste gas. From there it gets transported by the circulatory system to weak sites in the body where it causes various Vata diseases like arthritis, weight loss, insomnia, mental agitation and nervous system disorders.

Marma therapy is an important way of working on Prana, which governs our entire functioning. Prana in turn is connected to Vata dosha or the biological air-humor, which therefore is the most important of the humors in the development and treatment of disease. This makes marmas particularly important in dealing with Vata, which relates to deep-seated, chronic and degenerative diseases.

Depending on its site and function, Vata is divided into five types or *subdoshas*— Prana, Udana, Vyana, Samana and Apana. These are called the five Pranas, five Vatas or, more specifically, the five *Vayus* or airs. They are also important for the practice of Yoga and for the interface of Yoga and Ayurveda.

- *Prana Vayu* is responsible for the intake of nutrients that provide fuel for the body and mind, including food, water, air and impressions. Its main region in the body is in the region of the head and it is connected to the marmas located there. Prana Vata also has a special correspondence to the nerves.

- *Udana Vayu* is responsible for the upward movement of energy as in exhalation, speech, will and effort. Its main region in the body is the neck and it is connected to the marmas located there. Udana has a special correspondence with the muscles.

- *Vyana Vayu* is responsible for the outward movement of energy as in the extension of the limbs or the arterial flow of the blood. Its main region in the body is the chest, arms and hands and it is connected to the marmas located there. Vyana has a special correspondence with the ligaments.

- *Samana Vayu* is responsible for the inward movement of energy as in the contraction of the limbs and the venous flow of the blood. It facilitates the breaking down and digestion of food. Its main region in the body is the navel and digestive organs and it is connected to the marmas located there. Samana has a special correspondence with fat tissue.

- *Apana Vayu* is responsible for the downward movement as in the discharge of the feces, urine or menstrual fluid. Its main region of the body is the lower abdomen, legs and feet and it is connected to the marmas located there. As it governs Vata's site of accumulation in the large intestine, it is the main form of Vata for the treatment of disease in general. Apana has a special correspondence with the bones.

Of the five forms of Vata Dosha, marmas are most connected to Vyana Vayu, which governs the skin, circulation and the movement of Prana or vital energy. Therapeutic touch occurs mainly through Vyana, which distributes Prana throughout the body and can direct Prana as a healing force outside the body as well. Vyana also distributes the effects of herbs and oils through marmas to the rest of the body.

2. Pitta Dosha
The Principle of Digestion or Thermogenesis

- Pitta means 'that which cooks or digests things'. It is composed of the fire and water elements (with the oily aspect of liquids providing for its fuel in the body).

- Pitta is responsible for the conversion of food into heat, tissues and waste-materials. It governs digestion and metabolism from the cellular level to the tissue level, to that of the body as a whole. Its main physical disorders are fever, infection, inflammation and bleeding.

- At the mental level, Pitta is responsible for perception, judgment and determination and gives clarity and discrimination to the mind. Emotionally, Pitta creates drive and passion and its main disturbance is anger, which is toxic emotional heat or fire.

- Pitta's subtle or master form is called *Tejas* which provides positive warmth, radiance and insight. Tejas gives sexual vitality, courage and the ability to fight disease and resist cold.

- Pitta's main site in the body is the *small intestine*, where it accumulates in the form of acid and heat. From there it gets transported by the circulatory system to weak sites in the body and causes various Pitta diseases like ulcers, infections and inflammation of different types, particularly blood disorders.

Pitta dosha is divided into five types or subdoshas—*Pachaka, Ranjaka, Bhrajaka, Alochaka* and *Sadhaka*—which govern specific forms of digestion.

- *Sadhaka Pitta* is responsible for the digestion of nerve impulses by the brain. Marmas on the skull and brain generally relate to Sadhaka Pitta.
- *Alochaka Pitta* is responsible for the digestion of light through the eyes (and for digestion through the other senses). Marmas on the face and near the eyes relate to Alochaka Pitta.
- *Bhrajaka Pitta* is responsible for the digestion of sunlight and warmth through the skin. Marmas on the extremities and in the chest relate to Bhrajaka Pitta.
- *Pachaka Pitta* is responsible for the digestion of food through the digestive tract (particularly the small intestine). Marmas in the navel area relate to Pachaka Pitta. As it governs Pitta's site of accumulation in the small intestine, it is the main form of Pitta for the treatment of disease in general.
- *Ranjaka Pitta* is responsible for the coloring of the blood, the bile, the urine and the feces and works mainly through the liver. Marmas in the region of the liver relate to Ranjaka Pitta.

Marma therapy can increase or decrease heat in the body, directly impacting Pitta dosha. Marmas have a special connection to Bhrajaka Pitta which governs the skin and joints where most marmas are located. This means that Bhrajaka Pitta is usually the most important form of Pitta relative to marma therapy. The application of therapeutic touch, heat or the use of aromatic oils directly affects Bhrajaka Pitta and through it the other forms of Pitta.

3. Kapha Dosha
The Principle of Coherence or Cohesion

- Kapha means 'that which holds things together'. It is composed of water and earth elements, which are its states of motion (water) and rest (earth).
- Kapha is responsible for the formation of new tissue, for hydration, nutrition, lubrication and protection of the body against heat, wind, wear and tear. The body as a whole is composed mainly of Kapha (earth and water). Kapha's main physical disorders are accumulations of mucus, water or excess tissue development, particularly fat or adipose tissue.
- Psychologically, Kapha is the basis of feeling and emotion, love and caring. It imparts stability, calm and contentment to the mind. Emo-

tionally, its main disturbance is attachment, which results from too much heaviness (earth and water) in the mind.

- Kapha's subtle or master form is called *Ojas*, which is the essence of all the bodily tissues. Ojas is responsible for resistance to disease, endurance, strength, patience, fertility and longevity. Ojas provides the foundation for good health, emotional happiness and peace of mind.
- Kapha's main site in the body is the *stomach*, where it accumulates in the form of mucus or phlegm. From there it gets transported by the circulatory system to weak sites in the body and causes various Kapha diseases like asthma, diabetes, edema, heart disease and obesity.

Kapha's subtypes or subdoshas are called—*Tarpaka, Sleshaka, Avalambaka, Kledaka* and *Bodhaka*—which govern specific forms of lubrication.

- *Tarpaka Kapha* is responsible for lubrication of the brain and nervous system. It mainly relates to marmas on the head, skull, heart and spine.
- *Bodhaka Kapha* is responsible for lubrication of the tongue and sense organs in the head. It relates to marmas in the region of the head and face.
- *Sleshaka Kapha* is responsible for lubrication of the joints. It relates to marma points located in the joints and extremities.
- *Kledaka Kapha* is responsible for lubrication of the digestive tract. It relates to marmas in the region of the stomach.
- *Avalambaka Kapha* is responsible for lubrication of the heart and lungs. It relates to marmas in the chest region. As it governs Kapha's site of accumulation in the stomach, it is the main form of Kapha for the treatment of disease in general.

Marma therapy can be used to promote the circulation of Prana and break up accumulations of Kapha, which is increased by stagnation and lack of movement. As marmas are commonly connected to joints, they have a special association with Sleshaka Kapha.

Just as the doshas work together for creating health or disease, so do the subdoshas.

- Prana Vayu, Sadhaka Pitta and Tarpaka Kapha relate to the brain, spine and nervous system and the region of the head, along with the marmas in these areas.
- Udana Vayu, Alochaka Pitta and Bodhaka Kapha relate to the senses, face, mouth and neck, along with the marmas in these areas.
- Samana Vayu, Pachaka Pitta and Kledaka Kapha relate to the digestive

system, mainly the stomach and small intestines and Agni (digestive fire), along with the marmas in these areas.

- Vyana Vayu, Bhrajaka Pitta and Sleshaka Kapha relate to the skin, joints, extremities and surface of the body, along with the marmas in these areas.

- Apana Vayu, Ranjaka Pitta and Avalambaka Kapha relate to the internal organs of the lower abdomen, middle abdomen and chest, along with the marmas in these areas.

Marmas, however, do not affect only the doshic factors in their own region of the body, though this is an important consideration. They often have broader and indirect influences as well. Marmas on the extremities, for example, can strongly impact the internal organs and tissues of the body.

The Three Doshas and Individual Constitutional Types

Marma and Ayurvedic Constitution

Besides their general role within the body as a whole, the doshas imprint each one of us in a unique manner as our particular nature or type. Usually one dosha marks our individual mind-body or *Ayurvedic constitution* as a Vata, Pitta or Kapha predominant person.

- VATA TYPES are airy in their physical characteristics with a thin frame, low body weight, poor resistance to disease, and lack of tissue development. They easily overextend themselves and fall into conditions of exhaustion or debility. They are sensitive to wind, cold and dryness as environmental factors and feel better in conditions of warmth, moisture, rest and nurturing support. Psychologically, Vatas are restless, active, nervous and creative individuals, with many talents, who are often hypersensitive and can be a bit fragile.

- PITTA TYPES are fiery in their physical characteristics with a moderate frame, moderate body weight, strong appetite, ruddy complexion, good circulation and warm extremities. They easily overheat themselves and quickly come down with various infectious diseases. They are sensitive to heat and light as environmental factors and feel better in conditions of coolness and calm. Psychologically, Pittas are determined, intelligent, motivated and aggressive individuals who achieve their goals in life but often run into conflict.

- KAPHA TYPES are watery in their physical characteristics with a stocky frame, sturdy build and good tissue development. They dislike movement and easily accumulate weight, water or mucus owing to their slow metabolisms. They are sensitive to cold, dampness and stagnant air as environmental factors and feel better in conditions of warmth, dryness and increased activity. Psychologically, Kaphas are emotional, caring, stable and conservative types who value their feelings but easily get attached.

Mixed doshic types also occur, in which two doshas exist in relatively equal proportions as Vata-Pitta types, Pitta-Kapha types, or Vata-Kapha types. Occasionally, people may have all three doshas in relatively equal proportion (a Vata-Pitta-Kapha type). These doshic constitutions are the Ayurvedic *mind-body types* well-defined in general books on Ayurveda, which usually contain tests to help you determine what your type may be. Please examine such books for more information on this important topic.[3] Below is a typical Ayurvedic constitutional chart to help you determine your own constitution.

Ayurveda Constitution Chart			
	VATA (AIR)	**PITTA** (FIRE)	**KAPHA** (WATER)
HEIGHT:	tall or very short	medium	usually short but can be tall and large
FRAME:	thin, bony, good muscles	moderate, developed	large, well-formed
WEIGHT:	low, hard to hold weight	moderate	heavy, hard to lose weight
SKIN LUSTER:	dull or dusky	ruddy, lustrous	white or pale
SKIN TEXTURE:	dry, rough, thin	warm, oily	cold, damp, thick
EYES:	small, nervous	piercing, easily inflamed	large, white
HAIR:	dry, thin	thin, oily	thick, oily, wavy
TEETH:	crooked, poorly formed	moderate, bleeding gums	large, well-formed
NAILS:	rough, brittle	soft, pink	soft, white
JOINTS:	stiff, crack easily	loose	firm, large
CIRCULATION:	poor, variable	good	moderate
APPETITE:	variable, nervous	high, excessive	moderate but constant
THIRST:	low, scanty	high	moderate
SWEATING:	scanty	profuse but not enduring	slow to start but profuse

STOOL:	hard or dry	soft, loose	normal
URINATION:	scanty	profuse, yellow	moderate, clear
SENSITIVITIES:	cold, dryness, wind	heat, sunlight, fire	cold, dampness
IMMUNE FUNCTION:	low, variable	moderate, sensitive to heat	good, high
DISEASE TENDENCY:	pain	fever, inflammation	congestion, edema
DISEASE TYPE:	nervous	blood, liver	mucous, lungs
ACTIVITY:	high, restless	moderate	low, moves slowly
ENDURANCE:	poor, easily exhausted	moderate but focused	high
SLEEP:	poor, disturbed	variable	excess
DREAMS:	frequent, disturbed	moderate, colorful	infrequent, romantic
MEMORY:	quick but absent-minded	sharp, clear	slow but steady
SPEECH:	fast, frequent	sharp, cutting	slow, melodious
TEMPERAMENT:	nervous, changeable	motivated	content, conservative
POSITIVE EMOTIONS:	adaptability	courage	love
NEGATIVE EMOTIONS:	fear	anger	attachment
FAITH:	variable, erratic	strong, determined	steady, slow to change
TOTAL 30	**Vata____**	**Pitta____**	**Kapha____**

Marma Therapy and Doshic Types

Naturally the treatment of marmas must consider such constitutional factors. Marmas as energy centers are most connected with Prana and with the corresponding Vata dosha as already noted, but they have their effects on the other two doshas as well.

- VATA TYPES can use marma points to monitor and treat the level of Vata in their bodies and minds. They can benefit from marma therapy that aims at reducing Vata from its various places of accumulation in the large intestine, bones, joints and nervous system. Marma therapy can be used for pain relief, reducing stiffness, stopping tremors, relieving constipation, calming down anxiety, relieving stress, promoting sleep and other Vata-reducing actions.

- PITTA TYPES can use marma points to monitor and treat the level of Pitta in their bodies and minds. They can benefit from marma therapy that aims at cooling down high Pitta from its various places of accumulation in the small intestine, liver and blood. Marma therapy can be used for removing acidity, cleansing the blood, detoxifying the liver, countering infection, stopping inflammation, calming anger and other Pitta-reducing actions.

- KAPHA TYPES can use marma points to monitor and treat the level of Kapha in their bodies and minds. They can benefit from marma therapy that aims at moving and eliminating Kapha from its places of accumulation in the stomach and lungs, lymphatic system and fat tissues. Marma therapy can be used for reducing mucus, removing congestion, eliminating edema, promoting weight reduction, increasing physical and mental activity and other Kapha-reducing actions.

Other Bodily Factors

I. The Seven Tissues

To understand the body, we must understand the seven tissues that compose it. The tissues are called *dhatus* meaning 'prime constituents'. They are the main substances that do not get eliminated from the body (except for the reproductive secretions). They remain within the limit of the skin from the outside and the internal membranes of the organs and joints from within the body. The tissues go on developing throughout life. Their proper maintenance is essential for health and longevity. They are seven in number.

Name	Character	Function	Anatomical Counterpart
1. PLASMA *Rasa dhatu*	Plasma and mucous membranes	Nutrition	Skin
2. BLOOD *Rakta dhatu*	Hemoglobin portion of the blood	Oxygenation	Blood vessels
3. MUSCLE *Mamsa dhatu*	Muscle tissue	Movement	Muscles and internal organs
4. FAT *Meda dhatu*	Fat or adipose tissue	Lubrication & cushioning	Surrounding adipose formations
5. BONE *Asthi dhatu*	Bone tissue and cartilage	Support and protection	Bones and skeleton
6. NERVE *Majja dhatu*	Nerve tissue and bone marrow	Transmission of nerve impulses	Brain and spinal cord
7. REPRODUCTIVE *Shukra dhatu*	Reproductive tissue and secretions	Reproduction	Testes, uterus

Marma therapy works on the tissues of the body by increasing or decreasing the circulation through them. In this way, it primarily promotes the flow of blood and plasma. But marma therapy is also an important method of working on the deeper tissues of bone and nerve, the seats of Prana and Vata. This is because many marma points are on the head or on the joints, both of which connect directly to Prana and Vata.

The outer tissues of plasma and blood are affected mainly by nutrition, our daily intake and digestion of food and drink. The inner tissues of nerve and reproduction are affected mainly by our behavior, how we develop our minds and relate to other people. The intermediate tissues of muscle, fat and bone have a strong nutritional component but are also strongly affected by our behavior in terms of exercise and posture. Marma therapy can help us change behavioral patterns, though unlocking the Prana held in the deeper tissues. Even deep-seated psychological problems and addictions can be treated by marma therapy, which releases them from the joints, bones and nerve tissues in which they are held.

II. Waste-Materials

The waste-materials or *malas* are the constituents eliminated from the body during the normal course of metabolism. They vary from gaseous, liquid, semi-solid, to solid in form. The three main malas or gross waste-materials are urine, feces, and sweat. Proper elimination through the colon is essential for controlling Vata. Proper urination is important for controlling Pitta. Proper sweating is important for controlling Kapha.

In addition to these are subtle waste-materials (kleda) or exudations eliminated from the epithelial linings of the eyes, nose, mouth, ears and genital organs. Other minute waste-products are also formed during tissue formation and as a by-product of cellular metabolism.

The main tissue that relates to Kapha is the plasma (Rasa dhatu), which produces Kapha (mucus) as a waste-matèrial. The main tissue relative to Pitta is the blood (Rakta dhatu), which produces Pitta (bile or excess blood) as a waste-material. For this reason, most Kapha diseases involve the plasma and lymph glands and most Pitta diseases relate to the blood. The main tissue relative to Vata is bone (Asthi dhatu), which holds Vata in its joints and porous spaces. While Vata is not a waste-material of the bone, it is contained within the bones. Hence most Vata diseases, such as arthritis, involve the bones.

Health is maintained when waste-products are eliminated properly and in a timely manner. Certain marma points can be used to promote or inhibit their discharge from the body in order to normalize them.

III. Channel Systems

Ayurveda views the human body as composed of innumerable channels, like irrigation canals, which supply the nutrients to and remove waste materials from the various tissues. These channels are called *Srotas* in Sanskrit, from the root *sru* meaning 'to flow', with *Srotamsi* as the plural of the term. The channels are similar to the physiological systems of Western medicine.

Three channels connect the interior of the body to the outside environment, bringing in nourishment to the body in the form of breath, food, and water:

1. Respiratory System—*Pranavaha Srotas*

Pranavaha Srotas, the channels that carry Prana, the breath and vital force. It consists primarily of the respiratory system, though aspects of the circulatory and digestive systems are involved as well. It relates to the subtle or energy body (Pranamaya Kosha) which envelopes and gives life to the physical body.

This system has its origin in the heart and gastrointestinal tract since Prana is not only absorbed through the lungs but also is taken from food through the digestive tract and is distributed through the blood and plasma by the action of the heart. Many marma points work on this system because of their direct connection with Prana.

2. Digestive System—*Annavaha Srotas*

Annavaha Srotas, the channels that carry food (anna), mainly the digestive system. Its origin is in the stomach and the left side of body where most of the digestive tract is located. It is called *Mahasrotas* or 'great channel' as it is the main canal in the body, the gastro-intestinal tract.

It is the dominant system that governs the physical body, which itself is called *Annamaya Kosha* or the 'sheath made of food'. Many marma points work on this system because it is the main system governing the body.

3. Water-metabolism System—*Udakavaha* or *Ambhuvaha Srotas*

Udakavaha Srotas, the channels that carry (convey) water (udaka or ambhu), and regulate water-metabolism. Its origin is the soft palate and the pancreas. It does not possess a simple anatomical equivalent in Western medicine, but is like the fluid-absorbing aspect of the digestive system.

It governs the assimilation of water and water-containing foods, including the digestion of sugar. Diabetes is an important disease that relates to it. Certain marmas affect it, largely by stimulating the flow of fluids throughout the body.

Three additional channels connect the interior of the body to the outside environment and provide the elimination of the three main waste-materials from the body.

4. Sweating System/*Swedavaha Srotas*

Swedavaha Srotas, the channels that carry sweat or perspiration (Sweda). Its origin is fat tissue, from which sweat arises, and the hair follicles to which the sebaceous glands are connected. Certain marmas can be used to increase peripheral circulation and promote sweating, which is an important treatment for many diseases starting with the common cold.

5. Excretory System—*Purishavaha Srotas*

Purishavaha Srotas or the excretory system, the channels that carry the feces (*purisha*). Its origin is the colon and rectum, the organ of excretion. Certain marmas can be used to regulate elimination, either to relieve constipation or to stop diarrhea.

6. Urinary System—*Mutravaha Srotas*

Mutravaha Srotas or the urinary system, the channels that carry (convey) the urine (*mutra*). Its origin is the bladder and kidneys, the organs of urination. Certain marmas can be used to regulate urination.

In addition, there are seven channel systems, one for each of the seven tissues, as well as one separate channel for the mind and senses, making a total of fourteen channel-systems:

7. **Plasma, Lymphatic System—*Rasavaha Srotas***

8. **Blood, Circulatory System—*Raktavaha Srotas***

9. **Muscle, Muscular System—*Mamsavaha Srotas***

10. **Fat , Adipose System —*Medavaha Srotas***

11. **Bone, Skeletal System—*Asthivaha Srotas***

12. **Nerve, Nervous System—*Majjavaha Srotas***

13. **Reproductive, Reproductive System—*Shukravaha Srotas***

14. **Mind, Mental System—*Manavaha Srotas***

There are two more channels in women: the menstrual system or *Artavavaha Srotas* and lactation system or *Stanyavaha Srotas*. These are a subset of the reproductive system (Shukravaha Srotas) and not always counted separately.

Marmas function as trigger points for regulating the movement of energy through these channels. They are closely connected to the anatomical structures, organs and orifices through which these channels flow.

IV. Agni, the Power of Digestion

The key force responsible for the functioning of the body is *Agni* or the power of digestion. There are several forms of Agni or fire in the body. Most notable is the prime digestive fire or 'fire in the belly' (Jatharagni) which digests the food and beverages or earth and water elements taken in through the mouth. Working along with it are the 'five elemental Agnis (Bhutagnis) located in the liver, which are responsible for converting the digested food mass into appropriate forms of the five elements in the physical body.[4] In addition, each of the seven tissues has its own Agni or digestive power responsible for its specific metabolism called tissue Agnis (Dhatvagnis)—making thirteen forms of bodily Agnis in total.

The digestive fire, however, is not simply a material fire, but a pranic or electrical fire. It helps to energize the bioelectrical force of Prana to circulate through the fluids and tissues of the body. To create the proper fuel for this pranic fire, food must be broken down into a homogenous semi-liquid mass that is oily in nature. Only then can proper digestion occur. Agni, like a flame in the abdomen, burns using the fuel of this oily food mass, just as a ghee flame burns using ghee or a candle burns using beeswax.

The digestive fire or Agni is the key factor in health. When it is low or weak the power of digestion is impaired. The improperly digested food mass becomes a toxic substance in the digestive tract, called *Ama* in Sanskrit. Such toxins or Ama set in motion the disease process and invade the tissues and organs creating various ailments, minor or severe in nature. Various marmas can be treated for strengthening the digestive fire and for reducing Ama, aiding in its removal from the body.

In addition to the digestive fire, the breath itself is a gaseous or pranic fire (Pranagni) that promotes the proper movement of energy throughout the body. Various marmas can be used to increase Pranagni and keep our vital energy at its optimal condition and able to counter any disease attacks. This pranic nature of Agni makes it possible to work on it through pranic healing and marma therapy.

Each of the five senses also has its own Agni that aids in the reception and recognition of sensory impressions.[5] In the same way, the mind has its own Agni through which it digests emotions, ideas and experiences.[6] Certain marmas are special Agni points and can help catalyze these different forms of Agni, which are all interrelated. So whenever we think of marma points, we must consider both Prana and Agni.

---

[1] Note *Ayurveda, Nature's Medicine* (Frawley and Ranade) by the authors of this book.

[2] For example, commentaries on the *Hatha Yoga Pradipika*, a classical work on Yoga, lists the reduction of rajas and increase of sattva as one of the main goals of asana practice (I.17, Brahmananda commentary).

[3] Please consult books like *Ayurvedic Healing* (Frawley) or *Ayurveda, Nature's Medicine* (Frawley and Ranade) for more information.

[4] These are connected to Ranjaka Pitta that also works in the liver.

[5] These are connected to Alochaka Pitta which governs the eyes.

[6] These are connected to Sadhaka Pitta which governs metabolism in the brain.

CHAPTER 3

Marmas, Their Nature and Classification

The human body consists of an intricate network of channels, organs, circuits and tissues on many levels from the blood to the most refined nerve tissue of the brain. These interrelated channels create various patterns, linkages and interchanges across which substances, energy and information continually travel and circulate creating the mosaic of systems that makes up who we are.

The great ancient Ayurvedic teacher Sushruta described the constituents of the body in terms of 7 layers of skin, 300 bones (including cartilages and teeth), 210 joints, 900 ligaments, 500 muscles, 16 major tendons, 700 veins, arteries and nerves, and 107 marmas. This means that marmas are important identifiable parts of our anatomy and reflect key physiological and psychological processes that occur within it. As a surgeon, Sushruta stressed the importance of marmas in surgical practice. He stated that in any surgical procedure knowledge of marmas is as essential as knowledge of the nerves, muscles, bones and blood vessels.[1]

Charaka mentioned six major marma regions in the body—the head, neck, heart, bladder, *ojas* (endocrine system) and *shukra* (reproductive system). These are sometimes reduced to three main vital centers—bladder (lower abdomen), heart and head, which house our most important vital organs. Marmas, therefore, have a strong foundation in our anatomy and physiology.

All major Ayurvedic texts refer to the total number of primary marmas as 107,[2] while the total number of primary marma regions is 51. The difference between these two numbers is because several marmas exist on both sides of the body, and some marmas contain more than one marma point.

However, many Ayurvedic teachers recognize more marmas than these classical 107. Even Sushruta lists additional marmas beyond these.[3] Clearly there are more significant sites on the body than these 107. A number of these 'extra' marmas are mentioned at various places in this book (like the point in the center of the forehead or points by the *chakra* sites along the spine). In fact, every point on the body is potentially a marma point because the entire skin or surface of the body is itself a marma or sensitive region. One could say that the skin itself is the 108th marma, linking all the other marmas together.

As Vata and Prana are held in the joints, each joint can also be viewed as a potential marma region. Our internal organs have additional marma points, either directly connected to them or connected by reflex points that can affect them from a distance. On top of such universally shared marma points, each person will have his or her own unique sensitive points depending upon weight, frame, posture, diet, behavior and age. Therefore, we should not look at marmas in a rigid way, though the classical 107 marmas are a good foundation to start with. The same principles of marma therapy can be applied to the extra marmas as well.

The Three Doshas and Three Main Marma Sites

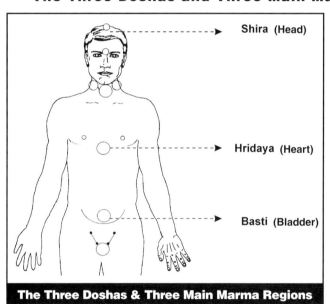

Shira (Head)

Hridaya (Heart)

Basti (Bladder)

The Three Doshas & Three Main Marma Regions

The three main marma regions—head, heart and bladder or lower abdomen—are the three main sensitive zones in the body. Although all organs and structures in the body can be related to all three doshas to some degree, the lower abdomen with its connection to the urinogenital and excretory organs relates more to Vata, the heart with its connection to the blood relates more with Pitta, and the head with its pool of nerve and brain tissue relates more to Kapha. As the doshas are the three main forces responsible for creating the entire body, marmas reflect their impact on our physiology in various ways.

Lethal and Therapeutic Marmas

Marmas are broadly classified into two categories as *lethal* or as *therapeutic* regions. Lethal marmas are points where the life-force can be hit and driven out of the body, causing injury, unconsciousness or even death. Therapeutic points are regions where the vital force can be treated for healing purposes. Lethal regions are areas which if struck or injured threaten the life of a person. Therapeutic regions are sensitive points that can be used to direct energy and counter diseases. Lethal areas, therefore, are more important for the martial arts, while therapeutic points are more significant for medical purposes.

Lethal marmas are often too sensitive for direct touch or manipulation. As regions like the throat, they can be inappropriate for stronger therapies like acupressure or acupuncture, but can be worked on in a limited manner if touched in a gentle way or if approached through pranic healing. Though not as significant for most healing purposes, they are important for diagnostic purposes as disease is often reflected in pain or dysfunction at their locations.

Therapeutic regions, like marmas on the arms and legs, are the most important for treatment purposes. They are easy to work on through procedures like massage, acupuncture, oils, aromas or ointments. However, these two types of marmas cross over to a great extent. Vulnerability can make an area important for therapeutic purposes. In addition, lethal areas often have therapeutic points around them that can be used while avoiding their more central vulnerable areas.

Physical and Energetic Definitions of Marmas

The concept of marma includes a whole range of anatomical structures like the skin, bones, joints, nerves and internal organs. Many marmas are on the limbs of the body, like those of the elbow and knee. We can easily work upon these *external marmas* through therapeutic touch. Some marmas like Shringataka (the soft palate) or Hridaya (heart) are located inside the body. These *internal* marma regions are best treated through reflex points above them on the surface of the body.

Marmas are defined anatomically according to their physical location. In this regard, the therapist should know the structures that define each marma and allow for its easy identification. However, we must not regard location of the marma as a simple physical phenomenon. Marmas are primarily 'energetic centers' where the life-force accumulates and flows. Treating them is more a means of treating Prana (the electricity running through the body) rather than simply working on physical tissues and organs (the light bulbs that carry the electricity). This is particularly true of larger marmas, like the knee (Janu marma) which have sensitive points in their vicinity that vary in location relative to the condition of the person.

This means that the main definition of marmas is not anatomical but energetic, in terms of Prana and the doshas. Their exact location depends upon the Pranas of both the therapist and the client, not simply on a fixed physical location. The patient should generally be treated where the Prana is focused in the marma region, which is not a fixed phenomenon. In addition, a good healer can direct his or her Prana to a marma region at almost any point within it. The Prana of a good therapist can easily find the weak or blocked Prana points on the client even without an extensive physical examination. *Prana will always work to heal Prana, just as water will naturally flow into low lying areas.* Therefore, the identification of marmas is an art and a matter of practice, not simply a physiological definition. This is one reason why exact marma locations may be slightly different according to different Ayurvedic practitioners.

Size of Marmas and Individual Finger Unit

Marmas are located and measured in size in terms of *anguli parimana* or the 'finger unit' of the respective individual. To determine this follow these instructions:

1. Join both open palms at ulnar (little finger) side.
2. Measure the width of both palms at metacarpo-phalangial joints (base of the fingers).
3. Divide this by 8 (as this width is average for 8 fingers).
4. This is individual finger unit.

Generally the height and breadth of a person is around 84 times the individual figure unit as shown in the illustration at left.

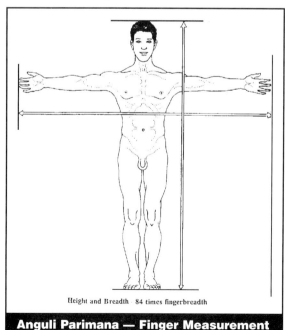

Height and Breadth 84 times fingerbreadth

Anguli Parimana — Finger Measurement

Marmas are classified according to their range in size as one-half finger unit (Anguli Parimana), one finger unit, two finger units, three finger units or four finger units (fist sized). Note *Appendix 3* for more information on this classification.

We can see from this classification that marmas vary greatly in size. While many marmas are as small as one-half finger unit in size, several like Hridaya (heart) marma are as large as four finger units. While smaller marmas can be called 'points', the larger marmas are more accurately described as 'regions' or 'zones'.

Marmas and Acupuncture Points

Marmas resemble acupuncture points in properties and usages. Sometimes they are referred to as 'Ayurvedic acupressure points'. However, we must be careful not to simply equate marmas and acupuncture points. Marmas can be much larger in size, are not always related to acupuncture meridians and are fewer in number than acupuncture points.

A pinpoint location of marmas is not always as crucial as for acupuncture points, particularly when marma treatment centers on massage rather than the use of needles (which Ayurveda rarely employs). So while recognizing the important similarities, we shouldn't confuse marmas with acupuncture points. The two can be very different.

Table of Marmas

Below is a table of the main marmas. As you can note, most marmas are named after their anatomical position, which in several instances occurs on both sides of the body. This list will serve as an introduction to how marmas are viewed. Note Part II of the book for a detailed description of each marma and note *Appendix 3* for a more detailed examination of the Sanskrit meaning of the marma name.

Marma	Location	Meaning	Size	Number
Adhipati	Top of the head	Overlord	½ unit	1
Amsaphalaka	Shoulder blade	Shoulder blade	½ unit	2, 1 on each side
Amsa	Shoulder	Shoulder	½ unit	2, 1 on each side
Ani (arm)	Lower region of the upper arm	The point of a needle	½ unit	2, 1 on each arm
Ani (leg)	Lower region of upper leg	The point of a needle	½ unit	2, 1 on each leg
Apalapa	Armpit or axilla	Unguarded	½ unit	2, 1 on each side
Apanga	Outer corner of the eyes	Looking away	½ unit	2, 1 by each eye
Apastambha	Upper side of the abdomen	What stands to the side	½ unit	2, 1 on each side
Avarta	Midpoint above the eyes	Calamity; from its sensitiveness	½ unit	2, 1 by each eye

Marma	Location	Meaning	Size	Number
Bahvi	Inside of upper arm	What relates to the arm	1 unit	2, 1 on each side
Basti	Lower abdomen	Bladder	4 units	1
Brihati	Broad region of the upper back	Wide or large	½ unit	2, 1 on each side
Guda	Anus	Anus	4 units	1
Gulpha	Ankle joint	Ankle joint	2 units	2, 1 by each ankle
Hridaya	Heart	Heart	4 units	1
Indrabasti (arm)	Center of forearm	Indra's arrow	½ unit	2, 1 on each arm
Indrabasti (leg)	Center of lower leg	Indra's arrow	½ unit	2, 1 on each leg
Janu	Knee joint	Knee joint	3 unit	2, 1 on each knee
Kakshadhara	Top of shoulder joint	What upholds the flank	1 unit	2, 1 on each shoulder
Katikataruna	Hip-joint	What rises from the hip	½ unit	2, 1 on each side of the back
Krikatika	Joint of the neck	Joint of the neck	½ unit	2, 1 on each side of the neck
Kshipra (hand)	Between thumb and index finger	Quick to give results	½ unit	2, 1 on each hand
Kshipra (foot)	Between big toe and second toe	Quick to give results	½ unit	2, 1 on each foot
Kukundara	On each side of lower iliac spine	What marks the loins	½ unit	2, 1 on each side
Kurcha (hand)	Bottom of thumb	A knot or bundle	4 units	2, 1 on each hand
Kurcha (foot)	Bottom of big toe	A knot or bundle	4 units	2, 1 on each foot
Kurchashira (hand)	Base of thumb joint	The head of kurcha	1 unit	2, 1 on each hand
Kurchashira (foot)	Base of big toe joint	The head of kurcha	1 unit	2, 1 on each foot
Kurpara	Elbow joint	Elbow joint	3 units	2, 1 on each elbow
Lohitaksha (arm)	Lower frontal end of shoulder joint	Red-jointed	½ unit	2, 1 on each arm
Lohitaksha (leg)	Lower frontal end of the hip joint	Red-jointed	½ unit	2, 1 on each leg
Manibandha	Wrist	Bracelet	2 units	2, 1 on each wrist
Manya	Side of upper neck	Honor	4 units	2, 1 on each side
Nabhi	Navel	Navel	4 units	1

Marma	Location	Meaning	Size	Number
Nila	Base of the throat	Dark blue	4 units	2, 1 on each side
Nitamba	The upper region of the buttocks	Buttocks	½ unit	2, 1 on each side
Parshva-sandhi	The upper hips	The side of the waist	½ unit	2, 1 on each side
Phana	Side of the nostrils	A serpent's hood	½ unit	2, 1 by each nostril
Shankha	Temple	A conch shell	½ unit	2, 1 on each side
Shringataka	Soft palate of the mouth	Place where four roads meet	4 units	4
Simanta	Fissures on the skull	Summit	4 units	5 on the skull
Sira Matrika	Base of the neck	Mother of the blood vessels	4 units	8, 4 on each side of the neck
Stanamula	Root of the breast	Root of breast	2 units	2, 1 on each side of the breast
Stanarohita	Upper region of the breast	Upper region of the breast	½ unit	2, 1 on each side of the breast
Sthapani	Point between the eyes	What gives support or fixes	½ unit	1
Talahridaya (hand)	Center of the palm of the hand	Center of the surface	½ unit	2, 1 on each hand
Talahridaya (foot)	Center of the sole of the foot	Center of the surface	½ unit	2, 1 on each foot
Utkshepa	Above the ears	What is upwards	½ unit	2, 1 by each ear
Urvi	The mid-region of the upper thigh	What is wide	1 unit	2, 1 on each leg
Vidhura	Behind and below the ears	Distress	½ unit	2, 1 by each ear
Vitapa	Perineum	What is hot or painful	1 unit	2, 1 on each side

Definitions of Marmas

There are several classical Ayurvedic definitions of marmas. From these we can see that marmas are related to the energies of the body, mind, Prana and doshas. They are key connecting points to all aspects of our energies from the inmost consciousness to the outermost physical organs.

1. Charaka defines marmas as sites where muscle, veins, ligaments, bones and joints meet together, though all these structures need not be

present at each marma. This explains marmas as important connection centers or crossroads in the physical body.

2. According to Vagbhatta, marmas are sites where important nerves come together along with related structures like muscles and tendons, a similar definition to that of Charaka. He says that sites which are painful, tender and show abnormal pulsation should also be considered as marma or vital points regardless of their anatomical structure. They are the seats of 'life' or Prana.[4] This means that any sensitive point on the body is a potential marma. Any injured area, for example, becomes a kind of marma point until it is healed.

3. According to Sushruta, marmas are places where the three doshas (Vata, Pitta and Kapha) are present along with their subtle forms as Prana, Tejas and Ojas and the three gunas of sattva, rajas and tamas.[5] This means that marmas control not only the outward form of the doshas, but their inward essences or master forms as well (Prana, Tejas and Ojas) and also the mind (sattva). Relating to Ojas or the power of immunity, marmas help maintain our immune system and can be treated in order to boost its powers. Connected to Ojas their treatment can be also used for rejuvenation. Connected to the mind, their treatment can relieve stress and promote meditation.

4. According to Dalhana, 'what can cause death if injured is a marma'.[6] While marmas do not always result in death, their impairment causes various diseases that can be difficult to treat.

5. Marmas mark the junction of the body with the mind, which is why we can feel pain when they are touched. They are important sites that can stimulate unconscious bodily processes, mental/sensory responses or emotional reactions. Treating them can release negative emotions and remove mental blockages, including those of a subconscious nature (like addictions). This means that there is an important psychological side to their treatment.

Composition of Marmas

Marmas are classified according to their dominant physical constituents as muscle, vessel, ligament, joint or bone-based regions. The descriptions below follow Sushruta, except for the last category of nerve. Note *Appendix 3* for more information on this classification.

1. Muscle-based Marmas (Mamsa Marmas)—related to muscle-based structures like facia, serous membranes, sheaths and muscles.

2. Vessel-based Marma (Sira Marmas)—related to various vessels or channels supplying energy or fluids to the body, particularly the blood and lymphatic vessels. Sushruta explains four types of these vessels:[7]

A) Vata-carrying Vessels (*Vatavaha Sira*), darkish in color. Vagbhatta says that impulses flow in this type of channels, connecting them with the nerves,[8] but they can also refer to energy carrying channels not entirely physical in nature.

B) Pitta-carrying Vessels *(Pittavaha Sira)*, yellowish in color, connecting them with heat, color (pigmentation factors), bile and lymph. They can also refer to smaller vessels carrying heat or enzymes.

C) Kapha-carrying Vessels (*Kaphavaha Sira)*, whitish in color, connecting them to lymphatic vessels, channels that carry mucus and other fluid or plasma-conveying channels.

D) Blood-carrying Vessels (*Raktavaha Sira)*. Vagbhatta says that they are deep-seated and carry red-colored blood, which would identify them with arteries and veins.[9]

Channels carrying the doshas are more energetic than anatomical in basis and so anatomical correlations are only general. Sushruta notes that no single vessel carries Vata, Pitta or Kapha alone. All vessels to some degree carry all three of the doshas, so their doshic distinctions are only general.

3. Ligament-based Marmas (Snayu Marmas)—related to the tissues and structures that bind the bones and muscles together. There are four types: ligaments proper, tendons, sphincter muscles and aponeuroses.

4. Bone-based Marmas (Asthi Marmas)—related to bony tissue, can be classified into bones proper, cartilage, teeth and nails.

5. Joint-based Marmas (Sandhi Marmas)—related to the joints, are important sensitive regions on the body for both Prana and the doshas. Joints are classified into movable, partially movable and non-movable. These can be complex or large marmas.

Symptoms of Injury to Marmas
Marmas are susceptible to damage from injuries, accidents, falls, wounds and other catastrophic events. Their injury results in bleeding, disorientation, loss of coordination, loss of consciousness and long term disability. It can affect all three doshas as well as the blood, Prana and the mind. Significant injury to marmas results in severe and often very special symptoms.

Vagbhatta notes, "When marmas are injured, a person rolls in bed due to pain, feeling as though entering into emptiness. He suffers from faintness and restlessness and has difficulty breathing. Due to severe weakness, he cannot lift his legs and hands, has a burning sensation in the heart, cannot stay in any posture for long and may soon succumb to death." [10]

The effects of injuries to marmas will vary according to the composition of the marmas. Any injury of a penetrating or lacerating type to a marma region will naturally produce hemorrhage and blood loss. If it occurs at a vessel (Sira) type marma (veins and arteries) like in the region of the neck, the blood loss can be severe. If a joint-based (Sandhi) marma is injured it will become difficult to move the joint, which may become swollen, reddish or distorted. Injury to a muscle-based (Mamsa) marma results in pain, paralysis, atrophy or edema of the muscle.

Five Types of Marmas Relative to Symptoms When Injured

Marmas are also classified according to five types relative to their degree of vulnerability. [11] These are *Sadya Pranahara* (Instant Death-Causing), *Kalantara Pranahara* (Long-term Death-Causing), *Vishalyaghna* (Fatal If Pierced), *Vaikalyakara* (Disability-Causing) and *Rujakara* (Pain-causing). This is a very important consideration that is defined in terms of the five elements. *However, the elements in this context do not reflect the dosha controlled by the marma but only the effects that occur if the marma is injured.* For example, marmas that govern the main heat centers in the body (bladder, navel and heart) are classified as fiery and are the most vulnerable, but these are not all primary Pitta sites. Please examine *Appendix 3* for more information on this important classification.

1. *Sadya Pranahara*—Immediate Death-Causing

Sadya Pranahara means 'immediately taking the Prana or life-force away', like the bursting of a balloon. They are sites where Prana can be quickly harmed and driven from the body. Significant injury to these marmas can prove fatal within twenty-four hours, and usually results in severe pain along with loss of consciousness. These marmas are key points of vitality like the heart, navel or bladder, said to be *fiery or heating in their degree of vulnerability*. When the heating power, bodily warmth and power of circulation which they control is weakened, our lives are immediately threatened. Injury to these main heat-holding marmas results in severe symptoms ranging from internal hemorrhage, coma, and irregular heartbeat (head and heart marmas), blood in urine, extravasation of blood or urine in peritoneal cavity (Basti marma), shock and pain. If the injury is serious, the person may not live long.

2. *Kalantara Pranahara*—Long-term Death-Causing

Kalantara Pranahara means 'taking the Prana or life-force away over time', like causing a leak in a vessel. They are points at which Prana can be removed from the body in the long-term. Significant injury to these marmas causes our Prana to gradually drain away and can prove fatal after a period of two weeks or more. Injury to such locations harms ones vitality in a significant but not immediately life-threatening manner. These marmas are said to be *both fiery and watery, or heating and cooling in their degree of vulnerability in nature*. Their fiery nature makes them vulnerable but their watery nature protects them, so harm to vitality from their injury is only in the long run. Such are points like Simanta (skull points) or points on the chest (Stanamula and Stanarohita) which are sensitive but have the protection of bones or muscles.

3. *Vishalyaghna*—Fatal If Pierced

Vishalyaghna (Fatal If Pierced) marmas can prove fatal if the point is pierced. Traditionally, it is said that if a foreign body or weapon becomes lodged at these points, it is life-threatening to remove it. This highlights the danger of damaging these points. These marmas are key points of vitality said to be *airy in their degree of vulnerability*. These are important Prana points on the head, like Sthapani (the point between the eyes) and so can cause severe pain or injury as well as disturb the mind. They hold and protect the life-force (Prana or Vata), but if punctured allow it to quickly leave the body, causing severe harm.

4. *Vaikalyakara*—Disability-Causing

Vaikalyakara (Disability-Causing) marmas, if injured, result in damage to the marma, harming the tissues, bones, nerves and vessels involved, but nothing that will threaten the life of the person. These marmas are said to be *watery or cooling in their degree of vulnerability*, which preserves and protects them. Injury to them results more in debility than in death and is not always so serious. These are mainly points on the arms and legs at a distance from the main vital organs and so injury to them cannot cause so much internal damage.

5. *Rujakara*—Pain-causing

Rujakara (Pain-causing) marmas result in recurrent or constant pain, depending upon the severity of the injury, which gets aggravated when the marma region is touched, moved or otherwise affected. These marmas are said to be both *airy and fiery in their degree of vulnerability*, which makes them sensitive and unstable and so results in severe pain and inflammation if injured. They are mainly sensitive joints like the wrists and ankles.[12]

Injury to Marmas and the Three Doshas

Vata, Pitta and Kapha increase at different marmas either according to external factors like injury or according to internal factors like wrong diet. When in a condition of excess at a marma, each dosha will manifest its characteristic symptoms. Understanding these, we can monitor the doshic imbalances at marma sites. Note the two sets of factors and symptoms below.

Factors that Increase the Doshas at Marma Sites

- VATA DOSHA is most likely to get disturbed by external injuries to marmas, particularly marmas that relate to nerves, bones or joints, or injuries that result in significant blood loss. External factors of cold, dryness and wind also cause Vata to increase at various marmas. Vata is disturbed at marmas owing to internal factors of weakness, tissue deficiency, nervous digestion or hyperactivity.

- PITTA DOSHA increases at marmas owing to internal factors of hyperacidity, fever, inflammation or toxic blood. External factors like overexposure to heat, fire, bright lights or caustic chemicals also cause it to increase.

- KAPHA DOSHA increases at marmas owing to internal factors of accumulation of weight, water (edema), mucus, congestion or lack of movement in the region. External factors like cold, dampness and stagnant air also cause it to increase.

Symptoms of Excess Doshas at Marma Sites

- IF VATA IS DISTURBED AT ANY MARMA, there will be severe pain not only at the marma site but in the entire body. Vata symptoms like fear, anxiety, tremors, constipation, nervous indigestion, insomnia and nervous agitation will increase.

Anti-Vata therapies like the application of heat, warm oil massage, or Vata-reducing herbs like ginger, calamus or ashwagandha will bring these symptoms down.

- IF PITTA GETS DISTURBED AT ANY MARMA, there will be feelings of heat, irritability and fever often extending to the entire body. Pitta symptoms like inflammation or bleeding at the marma point will combine with general Pitta symptoms like burning sensations, hyperacidity, loose stool, red eyes or intolerance to light.

Anti-Pitta therapies such as the application of cold (ice), cooling oils like coconut, and cooling herbs like sandalwood or rose will bring these symptoms down.

- WHEN KAPHA BECOMES INCREASED AT ANY MARMA, there will be swelling, accumulation of fluid (edema) and congestion. Overall Kapha symptoms will increase with possible feelings of heaviness, lethargy, cough, tiredness and dislike of movement.

Anti-Kapha therapies such as the application of heat, fasting, taking of hot spices like ginger and cayenne, or using warming aromatic oils like eucalyptus or ginger will reduce these symptoms.

---

[1] *Sushruta Samhita Sharira Sthana VI.30.*

[2] *Sushruta Samhita Sharira Sthana VI.3, Ashtanga Sangraha sh. 7.1, Ashtanga Hridaya sh.4.*

[3] *Sushruta Samhita Chikitsa Sthana VII.38* and *Sharira Sthana IX.12*, for example, mentions six additional marmas relating to reproductive system problems along with Guda and Basti marmas. These are called Sevani, Mutraseka, Mutravaha, Yoni, Antahphala srotas and Shukraharini.

[4] *Ashtanga Hridaya Sh. 4.37, Ashtanga Hridaya Sh. 4. 2, Sushruta Samhita, Sharira Sthana. 6.15.*

[5] *Sushruta Samhita, Sharira Sthana VI.35.*

[6] *Marayanti iti marmani (Dalhana).*

[7] *Sushruta Samhita, Sharira Sthana VII.6-18.*

[8] *Ashtanga Sangraha sh.6.4.*

[9] According to Gananath Sen, these can be again subdivided into *Aruna,* nerve (sympathetic), *Nila,* veins, *Rohini,* arteries, *Keshika,* capillaries, *Gauri,* lymphatic vessels and *Dhamani,* nerves (motor).

[10] *Ashtanga Sangraha S.sh7.26-27.*

[11] *Sushruta Samhita Sharira Sthana VI.16.*

[12] These five types of marmas also relate to different anatomical factors. According to *Sushruta Samhita, Sadya Pranahara* (Immediate Death-Causing) marmas are composed of all five factors of veins, ligaments, muscles, bones and joints. Those belonging to *Kalantara Pranahara* (Long-term Death-Causing) marmas are composed of only four factors. *Vishalyaghna* (Fatal If Pierced) types are composed of three factors. *Vaikalyakara* (Disability-Causing) sites are composed of two factors and only one factor is present in *Rujakara* (Pain-causing) sites. The more factors involved in a marma, the more dangerous injury to it is likely to be.

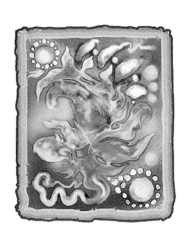

CHAPTER 4

Marmas
and the
Practice of Yoga

Yoga in its deeper sense is a spiritual science of Self-realization. Its aim is to lift our awareness to a higher consciousness that transcends pain and suffering, karma and rebirth. Toward this goal, the science of Yoga employs many practices and techniques. Asanas or Yoga postures work on our physical body to release stress, eliminate toxins and balance our physical energies. Asana is followed by internal methods of Pranayama (breath control) and Pratyahara (control of the senses) to calm and balance our vital energy and sensory impulses so that they do not disturb the mind. These, in turn, are followed by mantra and meditation to calm and balance the mind and make it receptive to higher influences.

Traditional Yoga reflects the physiological view of Ayurvedic medicine with its doshas, tissues and channel systems, including the role of marmas. Marmas are related to the chakra and nadi (subtle channel) systems emphasized in yogic thought. They are the focus of various Yoga practices, particularly those involving Prana. This is because marmas are important pranic centers. They also hold negative emotions and nervous tension (particularly Vata). Through working on marma points, we can control our Prana. Through Prana we can control our sensory and motor organs, and eventually the entire mind-body complex, affording us easy access to the higher realms of yogic consciousness.

Marmas, Chakras and Nadis

There are three levels of energy centers that link the body to the mind and higher consciousness—the chakras, the nadis and the marmas. The chakras are the energy centers of the subtle body that are located along the spine. They are the subtlest of the three, being of the nature of pranic or 'energy centers' rather than mere physical locations (which is why their actions are seldom perceptible at a physical level).

The nadis are the subtle channels that run from the chakras to various points on the body and which energize our physiological systems. They are not physical nerves but perceptible energy-flows.

Marmas are sensitive regions that develop from the nadis. They distribute the Prana from the chakras and the nadis throughout the body as a whole. They can be felt as certain points or zones on the body. Therefore, we can understand marmas as a development on a physical level of the energies that originate from the chakras and the nadis.

Three Types of Energy Centers

1. 7 Chakras
2. 14 Nadis
3. 107 Marmas

Marmas and the Seven Chakras

There are six main chakras or energy centers distributed along the spine as well as the seventh or main head center called the *Sahasrara* or 'thousand-petal lotus' that is connected to the brain. We should note that each of these chakras and its corresponding region of the back is a kind of marma or sensitive area. We could say that the chakras are the main marmas or pranic (energy) centers of the subtle body, which energize all the marmas or pranic centers of the physical body.

Chakra	Element, Sensory Quality, Sense Organ, Motor Organ	Nadis and Bodily Systems	Marmas
1. Muladhara, Root	Earth, Smell, Nose, Elimination	Alambusha Nadi, Excretory system	Guda (anus)
2. Svadhishthana, Sex	Water, Taste, Tongue, Reproduction	Kuhu Nadi, Urino-genital system	Kukundara, Vitapa
3. Manipura, Navel	Fire, Sight, Eyes, Feet	Vishvodhara nadi, Digestive system	Nabhi (navel)
4. Anahata, Heart	Air, Touch, Skin, Hands	Varuna nadi, Circulatory system	Hridaya (heart)
5. Vishuddha, Throat	Ether, Sound, Ears, Speech	Sarasvati nadi, Respiratory system	Nila, Manya, Amsa
6. Ajna, Third Eye	Mind, Inner Perception	Ida, Pingala, Pusha Gandhari, Payasvini Shankhini nadis, Nervous system	Sthapani, Apanga
7. Sahasrara, Head	Consciousness	Sushumna nadi, Brain	Adhipati, Simanta

We will not go into great detail about the chakras because this information is covered in many books.[1] However, we have presented their main factors of correlation relative to the marmas in a table below, including the elements, sense organs, motor organs, sense qualities, nadis, and bodily systems relative to each.

The important point to remember here is that *through treating their respective marmas, we can treat the nadis, elements, sense and motor organs, and other factors associated with the chakras*. For example, through treating the marmas in the region of the navel, one can work on the fire element in the body, including the digestive fire (Agni) and organs of the digestive system, the sense of sight and the feet as a motor organ. Relative to the nadis referred to in the table, these will be explained shortly.

Marmas and the Fourteen Nadis

Along with the seven chakras, the Yoga system emphasizes fourteen nadis or channels of the subtle body. Each nadi is identified by a point, aperture or orifice on the surface of the body that connects to it. All nadis begin at the root chakra or base of spine, move parallel to the Sushumna, which is the central nadi running up the region of the spine, and branch out from the Sushumna at various places. Apart from the Sushumna, the most important nadis are the Pingala and the Ida which, through the breath, govern the energy flow on the right and left sides of the body. Each nadi is connected to certain marmas. Through these marmas, we can treat the nadi and

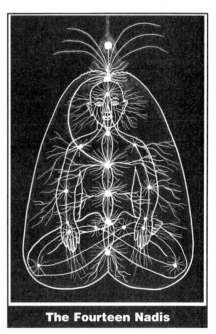

The Fourteen Nadis

insure the proper flow of Prana through it. Such nadi-marma points are very important.[2]

Nadis and the Chakras

Each chakra has a corresponding nadi that carries its energy to various portions of the body.

1. Alambusha nadi—Muladhara chakra

Extent	Runs from the center of the root chakra to the tip of the rectum. Supplies Prana to the organs of elimination.
Aperture	Aperture is the anus. Relates to the root or earth chakra and to Apana Vayu.
Marma	Corresponding marma is Guda (anus).

2. Kuhu nadi—Svadhishthana Chakra

Extent	Runs from the base of the spine to the sex chakra and forward to the end of the urethra. Supplies Prana to the urinary and reproductive organs.
Aperture	Aperture is the penis or vagina. Relates to the sex or water chakra and to Apana Vayu.
Marma	Corresponding marma is Basti (bladder).

3. Vishvodhara nadi—Manipura chakra

Extent	Runs from the base of the spine to the navel chakra and from it throughout the abdomen. Supplies Prana to the digestive system and digestive fire.
Aperture	Aperture is the navel. Relates to the navel or fire chakra and to Samana Vayu, Pachaka Pitta, Ranjaka Pitta and Kledaka Kapha. Supports the entire body through the digestive system and Agni.
Marma	Corresponding marma is Nabhi (navel).

4. Varuna nadi—Anahata chakra

Extent	Runs from the base of the spine to the heart chakra and from it throughout the entire body. Supplies Prana to the entire body, through the respiratory and circulatory systems and the skin.
Aperture	Aperture is the skin. Relates to the heart or air chakra and to Vyana Vayu, Bhrajaka Pitta and Avalambaka Kapha This nadi allows for the deeper feeling and knowing of the heart to manifest.
Marma	Main marma is Hridaya (heart), as well as other marmas in the chest.

5. Sarasvati nadi—Vishuddha chakra

Extent	Runs from the base of the spine to the throat chakra, branching out to the tip of the tongue. Supplies Prana to the throat, mouth, tongue and vocal organs.
Aperture	Aperture is the mouth and throat in general. Relates to the throat or ether chakra, to Udana Vayu and to Bodhaka Kapha. This nadi, as the name indicates, gives the powers of speech, song, taste, wisdom and mantra.
Marma	Corresponding marma is the tip of the tongue, which is not one of the classical 107 marmas. A reflex point for the Sarasvati nadi is in the middle of the jaw below the lips. Marmas in the throat region like Nila and Manya relate to it.

6. Sushumna nadi—Ajna chakra

Extent	Runs from the base of the spine to the top of the head, with many nadis branching out from it in the region of the third eye. Energizes the spine, the brain, the nerve tissue, and supports the bone tissue.
Aperture	Aperture is the eyes, specifically the point between the eyes or third eye. Collects and distributes the energy of all the nadis, particularly the eight right-left predominant nadis. Connected to Prana Vayu, Sadhaka Pitta and Tarpaka Kapha, Prana, Tejas and Ojas.
Marmas	Main marmas are Sthapani (third eye) and Adhipati (crown chakra).

Special Nadis for the Third Eye

The third eye or Ajna Chakra is the origin of six nadis that supply the senses, two for each of the nostrils, eyes and ears.

1. Pingala nadi

Extent	Branches out from the third eye, goes to the right nostril, which is its orifice, and supplies Prana to it. Also governs the right nasal passage.
Effects	Driving pranic channel for fiery and Pitta activities of all types from digestion to critical thinking. Also related to the root chakra which governs the sense of smell. Supplies en-

	ergy to the right side of the body, stimulating all the right side nadis.
Marma	Main marma is the right Phana marma.

2. Ida nadi

Extent	Branches out from the third eye, goes to the left nostril, which is its orifice, and supplies Prana to it. Also governs the left nasal passage.
Effects	Main Prana channel for watery and Kapha functions from tissue development to sleep. Governs inspired or visionary speech. Causes the whole body to be nourished through Prana. Also related to the root chakra which governs the sense of smell. Supplies energy to the left side of the body, stimulating all the left side nadis.
Marma	Main marma is the left Phana marma.

3. Pusha nadi

Extent	Branches out from the third eye, goes to the right eye, which is its orifice, and supplies Prana to it. Ruled mainly by Prana as the main power of the senses.
Effects	A very important nadi because the soul (Atman) dwells in the right eye during the waking state. Meditation upon the Seer in the right eye is a major approach to Self-realization in Yoga. Relates to Alochaka Pitta (the form of Pitta governing the eyes) and to the navel chakra, which governs the sense of sight.
Marma	Main marma is the right Apanga marma.

4. Gandhari nadi

Extent	Branches out from the third eye, goes to the left eye, which is its orifice, and supplies Prana to it.
Effects	Promotes dream, imagination and creative vision. Also relates to Alochaka Pitta and to the navel chakra which governs the sense of sight.
Marma	Main marma is the left Apanga marma.

5. Payasvini nadi	
Extent	Branches out from the third eye, goes to the right ear, which is its orifice, and supplies Prana to it. Also governs the right Eustachian tube.
Effects	At the right ear we hear the inner sounds of Yoga or *nada*, the music of the soul. Connected to the throat chakra which governs the sense of hearing.
Marma	Main marma is the right Vidhura marma.

6. Shankhini nadi	
Extent	Branches out from the third eye, goes to the left ear, which is its orifice, and supplies Prana to it. Also governs the left Eustachian tube.
Affects	Increases faith and makes us receptive to higher devotional influences. Also connected to the throat chakra which governs the sense of hearing.
Marma	Main marma is the left Vidhura marma.

The Two Nadis for the Arms and Legs

Two special nadis supply Prana to the right and left sides of the body and the arms and legs. Many different marmas occur in the field of these two nadis, which are very important for marma therapy. They relate to Vyana Vayu or the outward-moving vital air, though which our Prana radiates out and interfaces with the environment. They are connected to both the navel and heart chakras, which govern the hands and feet as motor organs and the flow of energy through them.

1. Yashasvati nadi	
Extent	Runs from root chakra to the navel chakra where it branches out. Supplies Prana to the right foot and right hand. Its energy comes to a center in the middle of the right hand and foot and from there radiates out to the five fingers or toes, ending primarily in the right thumb and big toe.
Aperture	Apertures are the tips of the right thumb and big toe.
Effects	There is a strong healing energy potential through the palm of the right hand, which like the right eye relates to

	the soul and to fire. Relates to Vyana Vayu, Bhrajaka Pitta and Sleshaka Kapha.
Marmas	Main marmas are Kshipra and Talahridaya on the right side of the body on both the hands and the feet. For all the marmas on the right side of the body, it is important to keep the energy flow in this channel clear and constant.

2. Hastijihva nadi	
Extent	Runs from the root chakra to the navel chakra where it branches out. Supplies Prana to the left foot and left hand. Its energy comes to a center in the middle of the left hand and foot and from there radiates out to the five fingers or toes, ending primarily in the left thumb and big toe.
Apertures	Apertures are the tip of the left thumb and big toe.
Effects	The energy of the left hand is more cooling, soothing and nourishing than that of the right and is watery in nature. This nadi relates to Vyana Vayu, Bhrajaka Pitta and Sleshaka Kapha.
Marmas	Main marmas are Kshipra and Talahridaya on the left side of the body on both the hands and the feet. For all the marmas on the left side of the body, it is important to keep the energy flow in this channel clear and constant.

Marmas and Yoga Practices

Marmas are an important factor to consider in regard to all Yoga practices from physical postures to Pranayama and meditation. They are an integral part of yogic thinking and the yogic understanding of both body and mind.

Marma and Asana Practice

One of the main purposes of the asana practice (Yoga postures) is to insure the right flow of Prana through the various marma regions. As many marmas are located in the joints, asanas help keep the marmas clear and energized. Therefore, it is important for an effective asana practice to consider the condition of the different marmic centers in the body, aiming at bringing better circulation to those marma regions that are stiff or tense. Marmas that are sore indicate the need to exercise the surrounding muscles and joints properly. Below are only a few suggestive indications as this is an important topic in itself outside the main scope of this book. Please examine specific works on Yoga asanas for more detail on the poses referred to.[3]

Sitting poses in general, but particularly the lotus pose (padmasana), serve to close and protect the marmas for the practice of meditation and for internalization of our energies of Prana and mind. The bound lotus (baddha-padmasana) in particular is a pose for locking and holding marma energy at an internal level.

Twists are excellent for unlocking marma energy generally, through improving the flow of Prana through the nadis, particularly for marmas in the back, hips and shoulders. Standing and extending poses (like trikonasana, virabhadrasana, parsvakonasana, or padangusthasana) serve to open and expand the marma system, connecting it with external sources of Prana and vitality.

Backward bends (like ustrasana and urdhva dhanurasana) generally open the marmas located on the chest and the front of the body and can strongly stimulate marma energy. Forward bends (like janu sirsasana, maricyasana and pascimottanasana) are better for marmas on the back of the body and are more calming to marma energy. Poses that bring the chest forward like upward facing dog and the cobra pose (urdhva mukhasvanasana and bhujangasana) are good for stimulating marmas in the chest.

Practices like *Uddiyana bandha* and *Nauli*, which aim at opening up the solar plexus, are excellent for marmas in the stomach region and for regulating Pitta in that area of the body. Practices like *Mulabandha*, which seal the energy in the root chakra, are excellent for marmas at the base of the spine and for regulating Vata in that area of the body. Practices like *Jalandhara bandha* and the more basic practice of *Ujjayi Pranayama* are excellent for marmas in the throat region and for regulating Kapha in that area of the body.

Inverted poses aid in the stimulation of marmas in the head and upper region of the body, depending upon the nature of the inversion. The headstand is very powerful for marmas in the head. The shoulder stand is excellent for marmas in the neck. Naturally, one must prepare for these poses properly, particularly for the headstand.

Marmas, Pratyahara and Pranayama

Marmas as pranic centers can be easily affected through Pranayama. Through Pranayama or yogic breathing we increase the flow of Prana through the chakras, nadis and marmas. Most notable in this regard is the practice of 'alternate-nostril breathing'. We can use the right nostril breathing (breathing in through the right nostril and out through the left), which is heating in nature, to energize the marmas on the right side of the body. We can use left nostril breathing (breathing in through the left nostril and out through the right), which is cooling in nature, to energize the marmas on the left side of the body. Another method is to use *Bhastrika Pranayama* to open the marmas in the region of the head.

Yet perhaps the main aspect of Yoga practice that actively considers the use of marmas is Pratyahara, the fifth of the eight limbs of Yoga. Pratyahara mediates between the outer factors of Yoga—specifically Asana that works upon the physical body—and the inner factors of Yoga—specifically Dhyana or meditation that works upon the mind. Pratyahara is the door between the outer and inner aspects of Yoga that allows us to turn our energy inward. Its role is crucial in taking Yoga practice from a mere physical exercise to a true spiritual discipline. Pratyahara is placed between Pranayama or pranic energization, the fourth limb of Yoga, and to *Dharana* or mental concentration, the sixth limb of Yoga. It serves to take the Prana inward, which frees it for both spiritual and healing purposes.

Pratyahara literally means 'withdrawal', like a turtle withdrawing into its shell. It refers to various internalization exercises designed to control the senses and motor organs and introvert the mind. Such Pratyahara practices include closing the eyes and ears to look and listen to the inner lights and sounds within and *mauna*, the practice of silence or not speaking in order to control the vocal organ. Common physical forms of Pratyahara consist of relaxation exercises—tightening and releasing the energy in various muscles and joints, which affects related marmas. This clears the energy in the organs and system that the marmas control.

We can understand the relevance of marmas and Pratyahara when we consider the marmas as 'pranic control points', through which Prana and the various organs of the body can be influenced. Each marma has corresponding organs, systems, senses, nadis and chakras that it rules over. Through working on the particular marma, we can control or affect these factors in various therapeutic ways.

The great yogic text, *Vasishta Samhita,* contains an important section explaining the use of specific marmas for the practice of Pratyahara. It states, "Great yogis ever praise Pratyahara as concentration (Dharana) on the eighteen marma places that hold Prana. Drawing the Prana from each of these places is said to be the best form of Pratyahara." We have included a translation and summary of the material as it is not available in English.[4]

The Eighteen Yogic Marma Regions and Corresponding Marmas

1. Toes   Kshipra marma
2. Ankles   Gulpha (ankle) marma

3. Middle of the calf	Indrabasti marma
4. Root of the knee	Not a classical marma, but can also be used
5. Center of the knee	Janu marma
6. Middle of the thigh	Urvi marma
7. Anus	Guda marma
8. Middle of the hip	Kukundara and Nitamba marmas
9. Root of the urethra	Vitapa marma
10. Navel	Nabhi (navel) marma
11. Center of the heart	Hridaya (heart) marma
12. Base of the throat	Nila marma
13. Root of the tongue	Shringataka marma
14. Root of the nose	Not a classical marma, relates to Phana marma by the nostrils
15. Center of the eyes	Apanga marma
16. Middle of the brows	Sthapani marma
17. Center of the forehead	Not a classical marma, but is still very useful.
18. Top of the head	Adhipati marma

These eighteen marma regions include points for seven chakras—the root of the anus (Muladhara), the root of the urethra (Svadishthana), the navel (Manipura), the heart (Anahata), the root of the throat (Vishuddha), the middle of the brows (Ajna) and the top of the head (Sahasrara). The regions of the eyes, the root of the nose, the root of the tongue, and the middle of the brows relate to the third eye or Ajna chakra as well. The point on the forehead also relates to the crown chakra.

These marma regions also relate to the fourteen nadis. The root of the anus relates to Alambusha nadi. The root of the urethra relates to Kuhu nadi. The navel relates to Vishvodhara nadi. The heart relates to Varuna nadi. The root of the tongue relates to the Sarasvati nadi. The top of the head relates to the Sushumna nadi. The root of the nose relates to Ida and Pingala nadis. The point between the eyes relates to the Pusha and Gandhari nadis. The marmas along the legs relate to the Hastijihva (left side) and Yashasvati (right side) nadis.

Marma Meditation

Below is a marma meditation using marma points according to this yogic teaching. *Vasishta Samhita* states, "One should practice concentration by drawing one's Prana by the power of attention from each of these marma regions."[5] To do this practice the following method carefully, using inhalation and exhalation at each marma region, much like flexing and relaxing of the muscles.

1. Direct your attention to your toes. On inhalation, gather your energy there. On exhalation, release it. Feel your toes energized, healed and relaxed.

2. Move your attention to your ankles. On inhalation, gather your energy there. On exhalation, release it. Feel your ankles energized, healed and relaxed.

3. Move your attention to the middle of your calves. On inhalation, gather your energy there. On exhalation, release it. Feel your calves energized, healed and relaxed.

4. Move your attention to the base of your knees. On inhalation, gather your energy there. On exhalation, release it. Feel the base of your knees energized, healed and relaxed.

5. Move your attention to the middle of your knees. On inhalation, gather your energy there. On exhalation, release it. Feel the middle of your knees energized, healed and relaxed.

6. Move your energy to the middle of your thighs. On inhalation, gather your energy there. On exhalation, release it. Feel your thighs energized, healed and relaxed.

7. Move your energy to the root of your anus. On inhalation, gather your energy there. On exhalation, release it. Feel your anus energized, healed and relaxed.

8. Move your energy to the middle of your hips. On inhalation, gather your energy there. On exhalation, release it. Feel your hips energized, healed and relaxed.

9. Move your energy to the root of your urethra. On inhalation, gather your energy there. On exhalation, release it. Feel your urethra energized, healed and relaxed.

10. Move your energy to your navel. On inhalation, gather your energy there. On exhalation, release it. Feel your navel energized, healed and relaxed.

11. Move your energy to your heart. On inhalation, gather your energy there. On exhalation, release it. Feel your heart energized, healed and relaxed.

12. Move your energy to the root of your throat. On inhalation, gather your energy there. On exhalation, release it. Feel your throat ener-

gized, healed and relaxed.

13. Move your attention to the root of your tongue. On inhalation, gather your energy there. On exhalation, release it. Feel your tongue energized, healed and relaxed.

14. Move your attention to the root of your nose. On inhalation, gather your energy there. On exhalation, release it. Feel your nose energized, healed and relaxed.

15. Move your attention to your eyes. On inhalation, gather your energy there. On exhalation, release it. Feel your eyes energized, healed and relaxed.

16. Move your attention to the point between your brows. On inhalation, gather your energy there. On exhalation, release it. Feel your brows energized, healed and relaxed.

17. Move your attention to the middle of your forehead. On inhalation, gather your energy there. On exhalation, release it. Feel your forehead energized, healed and relaxed.

18. Move your attention to the top of the head. On inhalation, gather your energy there. On exhalation, release it. Feel the top of your head energized, healed and relaxed.

In this practice, you should concentrate both your mind and Prana in each of these eighteen regions starting with the feet. Gather your attention from one marma region to another like climbing a series of steps from the bottom to the top of the body. Finally, hold your awareness at the top of the head in the space of the Supreme Self beyond birth and death and all suffering. In addition, you can also direct your attention to any of these marma sites individually in order to heal the area or for specific therapeutic purposes.

Marma and the Use of Mantra

Besides their usage for spiritual and yogic purposes, mantras have a wide application for healing purposes. Mantra therapy or *Mantra Chikitsa* is commonly used in all branches of Ayurveda and considered one of the most important Ayurvedic therapies for all types of diseases. Mantras facilitate the flow of Prana through the marma points and are another important tool of marma therapy.

Mantras have a special application to protect marma points. They can create a protective covering or armor, called 'kavacha' in Sanskrit, at a psychic or pranic level to shield various marmas. Many meditational kavachas have been designed for this purpose, using certain mantras or names of God to protect the vulnerable parts of the body. Kavachas are common in

Tantric texts where they occur in a great variety. Another practice is that of *nyasa* or consecration, where various parts of the body like the heart and forehead are touched with the hands along with the recitation of mantras in order to dedicate those areas to the deity. This is another important tool both of ritual and psychic healing.

For the sake of brevity and simplicity we will discuss only a few simple mantras. These are among the most energetically powerful as well as the easiest mantras to use. The *Mantra Purusha,* which correlates the fifty root sounds of the Sanskrit alphabet to the various parts of the body, can also be used for this purpose, if one wants to be more specific.[6]

Important Bija (Seed) Mantras and Usage with Marmas

- The mantra HUM (pronounced 'hoom', rhyming with room) is *Varma bija*, the seed sound of protection, possessing a fiery and wrathful nature. It is used specifically to protect marma points and is the most important mantra in this regard. The mantra HUM can be repeated relative to any marma that one wants to protect from injury or from energy loss. It can be used along with the marma meditation practice outlined above to create a protective field of mantra (mantra-varma) around the physical body and the aura. Visualize this mantra as creating a deep blue protective force that can ward away all negativity, disease or debility. Chanted with a shorter u-sound, as in the word 'put', HUM has a more fiery energy for purposes of warming the marmas and increasing Agni or fire at their locations.

- The mantra OM is *Prana bija* or the seed sound of energy and vitality. It can be repeated relative to any marma one wants opened, cleared and released. It carries the immortal force of the higher Self (Atman) and is expansive and ascending in its effects. Usually it is visualized as golden in color and as carrying a solar force of life and intelligence.

- The mantra AIM (pronounced 'I'm') is *Guru bija*, the seed sound of speech, guidance and concentration. It can be used for directing mental energy and healing intentions to any marma point. It holds the Sarasvati energy, the energy of knowledge, wisdom and creativity, and is white in color.

- The mantra KRIM (pronounced 'kreem') is the seed sound of *Kriya shakti*, the power of action and represents electrical or lightning force. It can be used to stimulate and energize any marma with pranic power. It holds the Kali energy, the energy of transformation, internalization and spiritual awakening, which is also the power of Yoga, and is dark blue in color.

- The mantra SHRIM (pronounced 'shreem') is the seed sound of harmony and well-being and projects a nutritive lunar energy. It can be used to heal or soothe any marma region, particularly from conditions of weakness or tissue depletion. It holds the Lakshmi energy or the positive force of health, creativity, happiness and prosperity.

- The mantra HRIM (pronounced 'hreem') is the seed sound of the heart, space and Prana and projects a solar force and golden color. It can be used to open, energize and heal any marma, particularly internal marmas like those of the heart. It holds the Goddess energy in general as a force of health, vitality and enlightenment.

- The mantra KLIM (pronounced 'kleem') is the seed sound of desire, attraction or magnetic energy, and projects the power of love. It can be used to increase Kapha or Ojas energy at any marma, including strengthening reproductive functions.

How to Use These Mantras

Choose any one of these mantras that you find suitable to work with. Chant it for a minimum of 108 times (or multiples thereof) for one month (preferably the period between two new moons). Meditate upon the marma you are focusing on and repeat the mantra along with the breath, energizing the marma on inhalation and releasing or expanding it on exhalation. For example, mentally repeat the mantra HUM on inhalation while visualizing the marma filling with a protective force, while on exhalation spread that protective force from the marma to around the body as a whole.

One can also use these mantras relative to the eighteen marma regions mentioned above. A good method is to use the mantra OM on inhalation in order to gather energy in the marma region, and the mantra HUM on exhalation to protect and fortify the marma. One can visualize OM as creating a golden light to energize the marma and HUM creating a dark blue light to protect it.

Mantras for the Five Elements

The body can be divided into five regions relative to the five elements. We can treat the elements in the body according to the marmas in the portion that relates to them.

1. MARMAS IN THE REGION FROM THE FEET TO THE KNEES BELONG TO THE EARTH ELEMENT.
   Key marma: Talahridaya on the feet.
   Key mantra: LAM (pronounced lum as in 'lump').

2. MARMAS IN THE REGION FROM THE KNEES TO THE
   ANUS BELONG TO THE WATER ELEMENT.
   Key marma: Urvi marma on the middle of the thighs.
   Key mantra: VAM (pronounced vum as in 'vulnerable').

3. MARMAS IN THE REGION FROM THE ANUS TO THE
   HEART BELONG TO THE FIRE ELEMENT.
   Key marma: Nabhi (navel) marma on the navel.
   Key mantra: RAM (pronounced rum as in 'rump').

4. MARMAS IN THE REGION FROM THE HEART TO THE
   MIDDLE OF THE EYEBROWS BELONG TO THE AIR
   ELEMENT.
   Key marma: Phana marma on the nostrils.
   Key mantra: YAM (pronounced yum as in 'yummy').

5. MARMAS IN THE REGION FROM THE MIDDLE OF THE
   BROWS TO THE TOP OF THE HEAD BELONG TO THE
   ETHER ELEMENT.
   Key marma: Adhipati marma on the head.
   Key mantra: HAM (pronounced hum as in 'hump').

The seed mantras of the five elements can be used to treat the marmas in their respective regions of the body. One can use the seed sound of Earth LAM to strengthen marmas on the feet like Talahridaya marma. One can use the seed sound of Water VAM to strengthen marmas on the thighs like Urvi marma. One can use the seed sound of Fire RAM to strengthen marmas in the middle of the body like Nabhi marma (navel). One can use the seed sound of Air YAM to strengthen marmas in the chest and throat like Hridaya marma (heart). One can use the seed sound of Ether HAM to strengthen marmas in the head like Adhipati marma.

Another method is to use the seed sounds of the elements in order to increase the element required to heal any marma. For example, if one wants to increase the fire element in the navel to stimulate the power of digestion, use the mantra RAM. If you want to increase the water element in the navel for countering acidity, use the mantra VAM.

You can also use these mantras along with alternate nostril breathing. For example, the mantra RAM can be repeated upon inhalation through the right nostril to increase the fire element on the right side of the body. Similarly, the mantra VAM can be used along with exhalation through the left nostril to increase the water element on the left side of the body. Or one can use the mantra HAM with alternate nostril breathing to increase the ether element in the entire body. In this way one can direct the energies of the five elements to either or both sides of the body and their corresponding sensory and motor organs.

Marmas, Color and Gem Therapy

The use of colors and gems is another important part of both yogic and Ayurvedic healing, particularly relative to Tantra and its energetic practices that work to harness the secret forces of nature. Gems are specifically referred to as *Mani* and provide one of the three main factors of Ayurvedic healing along with herbs and mantras. While some Ayurvedic doctors today who are trained in modern medicine may not use it, many traditional Ayurvedic practitioners as well as followers of energetic healing in the West find great value in these subtle therapies. Color and gem therapy can be used on marmas. Light is able to stimulate marmas in various ways depending upon its source and its color.

Marmas and Color Therapy

Colors can be applied with colored lamps, preferably projecting a focused ray on the general extent of the marma to be treated. Color can be used internally through visualization as well, meditating on the color as pervading the marma region. This can be combined with breath work (breathing the color into the marma). Special machines also exist for transmitting light through gemstones. These give a particularly high quality healing power to color therapy. Generally the marma should be bathed in the appropriate colored light for at least fifteen minutes for it to have an effect.

NOTE: in the chart below; P = Pitta, K = Kapha, V = Vata

DEEP BLUE
Energetics: PK-V+, increases Prana
Good for removing inflammation, infection and fever, and for stopping bleeding, also affords protection.
RED
Energetics: KV-P+, increases Agni
Good for stimulation, energization, warming, improving blood flow.
ORANGE/ SAFFRON
Energetics: VK-P+, increases Agni and Tejas
Good for energization, stimulation, warming, purifying and cleansing. Opens the mind.

GOLD
Energetics: VK-P+, increases Tejas and Ojas
Good for energization, pain relief, stimulation, and spiritualization, also promotes growth the tissue development. Transmits a solar force.

YELLOW
Energetics: KV-P+
Good for balancing, clearing, nourishing and grounding energy.

GREEN
Energetics: PK-V+, increases Prana
Good for giving vitality, promoting Prana, cleansing the blood, calming the nerves, balancing the mind and stopping pain.

WHITE
Energetics: PV-K+, increases Ojas
Good for balancing, nurturing and increasing tissues and bodily fluids (Kapha).

Marmas and Gem Therapy

Gem Therapy is called *Mani Chikitsa* in Sanskrit and is commonly used along with both herbal and mantra therapies. Gemstones provide a strong form of color therapy, working on a subtle level to help balance the flow of Prana and connect us with cosmic light sources that emanate from the stars and planets.

The Use of Crystals

Crystals are easy to use for marma therapy. They are not expensive and can be found in sufficient size (ten or more carats) to have a good effect. Polished stones are not necessary, though they can be more effective. A crystal can be placed on one marma, while the practitioner is working on another. A simple method is to tape the crystal on the respective marma, using a soft tape that doesn't damage the skin. Placing larger crystals on large marma regions like the heart or navel is another method. One can use the point of a crystal to stimulate a marma point, and the flat face of the crystal to calm it.

CLEAR CRYSTAL
Useful in clearing, energizing and opening marmas, making them receptive to healing forces.
MILKY CRYSTAL
Has a nourishing, moistening and calming lunar energy. Builds tissues and increases bodily fluids.
ROSE CRYSTAL
Warms, energizes and stimulates the circulation at marmas. Strengthens the blood.
CITRINE
Strengthens, tonifies and builds energy in marmas. Improves vitality and immune response.
AMETHYST
Cools, cleanses, purifies and detoxifies marmas. Good for acute pain or infection.

Primary Gems

For these stones, cut gems are preferable, which can be expensive. Uncut or unset stones can be used but may not be as strong in their affects. Cut gems can be used in small sizes, but should generally be at least one carat in size. Uncut stones should be used in larger sizes, preferably over five carats. Like crystals they can be temporarily taped over marma points. Or the therapist can hold the gem on the marma point using his thumb or middle finger for a minute or two.

However, it is more effective to keep such primary gems on marma points for a period of a month or longer for stronger action. Some marmas like those on the hands, arm, neck or heart can be treated by wearing rings, bracelets, bangles or pendants which touch them. For this it is best to have an open setting for the gem in which the gem can directly touch the skin. Such a 'marma-based gem therapy' is an important consideration whenever prescribing the use of gems.

Substitute stones to these primary expensive gems can be used much like the crystals mentioned above. The usage of primary gemstones is defined astrologically according to the rules of Vedic astrology (Jyotish), which can be examined for more information on the subject.[7] Such gems usually require an examination of the birth chart and should not be prescribed according to Ayurvedic indications alone.

NOTE: in the chart below; P = Pitta, K = Kapha, V = Vata

RUBY
Substitutes: red garnet, sunstone
Energetics: KV-P+, Increases Agni and Tejas
Transmits a powerful solar force to warm and stimulate marmas, promoting circulation, energy flow and relieving pain, strengthening the heart.

PEARL
Substitutes: moonstone, milky crystal, cultured pearls
Energetics: PV-K+, increases Ojas
Transmits a gentle lunar force to cool, lubricate and nurture marmas, countering dryness and debility, strengthening the lungs and soothing the emotions.

RED CORAL
Substitutes: carnelian
Energetics: P+(slightly) VK-, increases Ojas and Tejas
Transmits a Mars force to warm, strengthen and energize marmas. Helps build the blood, muscles and bone and improves male energy.

EMERALD
Substitutes: peridot, jade, green tourmaline
Energetics: VPK=, generally balancing, increases Prana
Transmits a Mercury or pranic energy to relieve pain and tremors, and counter mental or nervous agitation at marmas, calming for children. Helps heal injured marmas.

YELLOW SAPPHIRE
Substitutes: topaz, citrine
Energetics: VPK=, generally balancing, increases Ojas
Transmits a Jupiter energy to fortify, tonify and build good quality tissue at marmas, promoting vitality and longevity. Good for Ojas. Per-

YELLOW SAPHIRE Continued
haps the best strengthening stone for general usage, particularly good for the elderly.

DIAMOND
Substitutes: white sapphire, zircon, clear quartz crystal
Energetics: PV-K+, Increases Ojas
Transmits a Venus energy to clear, energize, and strengthen marmas, bringing the energy of Ojas (higher Kapha force) to them. Also improves female energy and strengthens the bones.

BLUE SAPPHIRE
Substitutes: amethyst, turquoise, lapis lazuli
Energetics: PK-V+
Transmits a Saturn energy to cool, cleanse, detoxify and calm the energy at marmas. Helps heal injured marmas, inhibiting bleeding and stopping infection.

Sacred Stones and Yantras

Other special stones can be used to heal marmas as well. One can use *Shivalingas* (Shiva stones) or *Shaligramas* (Vishnu stones), special small egg shaped rocks from rivers and mountains in India. These also help stabilize and heal marma points. For this purpose, small stones can be used of one to three inches in size. Or you can use any sacred stones that you may have. The important thing is that you are connected to the healing power of the stone. The Earth energy of such stones is very good for bringing calm and stability to pranic energy through the marmas. They are particularly good for countering

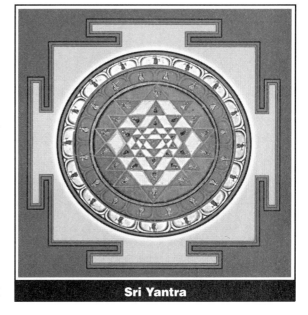

Sri Yantra

Vata dosha. They help conduct the healing energy from the Earth which in turn is connected to that of the stars and planets.

Another method is to place small *yantras* on marmas. Yantras are metal plates—usually made with copper but also with silver, gold or various alloys—that contain geometrical designs, mainly triangular in nature, along with inscribed mantras. Yantras serve as conductors for spiritual and cosmic energies. *Surya Yantra*, dedicated to the Sun, which represents Prana, is important in this respect. It consists of a six-pointed star with a circle in the middle along with various inscribed mantras for the Sun. Another important healing yantra for marma therapy is the *Sri Yantra* sacred to the Goddess, which consists of five upward facing and four downward facing triangles. It can be used with the mantras HRIM or SHRIM.

Such yantras are often available where Ayurvedic, Vedic astrology or Puja supplies are sold. Generally one should use small yantras of one or two inches in size for treatment purposes, energizing them with the appropriate mantras. These are most commonly found made out of copper which is a good metal for conducting pranic energy.

---

[1] Note *Yoga and Ayurveda* (Frawley) chapter 10 for more information on the chakras.

[2] Note *Yoga and Ayurveda* (Frawley) chapter 11 for more information on the nadis.

[3] Note Yoga for *Your Type: An Ayurvedic Approach to Your Asana Practice* (Frawley and Kozak).

[4] *Vasishta Samhita IV.57-75* for description of Pratyahara on eighteen marma regions.

[5] *Vasishta Samhita IV.61*

[6] Note *Yoga and Ayurveda* (Frawley) chapter 17 for information on the Mantra Purusha and the use of mantras.

[7] Note *Astrology of the Seers* (Frawley) chapter 14 for information on use of gems in Vedic astrology.

CHAPTER 5

The Many Methods of Marma Therapy 1: Massage, Aroma Therapy and Pranic Healing

Ayurvedic therapy combines all factors of right living, outwardly and inwardly, as well as every type of healing modality for body, mind and Prana. It is perhaps the world's most comprehensive and integral healing system, going to the roots of our being on physical, psychological and spiritual levels, and our connections with the greater universe of consciousness in all these areas.

Broadly speaking, Ayurvedic therapies can be divided either into 'methods for treating disease', applied mainly in a clinical setting, or 'health maintenance methods' that we can do on our own as part of a harmonious life-style. While marma therapy is part of Ayurvedic clinical treatments, aspects of it can be safely used as part of self-care, for treating ourselves, our friends or our family members.

Ayurvedic methods for treating disease are classified into two groups: those for removing toxins and reducing excess tissues, which are called 'reduction methods' (Langhana); and those for restoring vitality and rebuilding deficient tissues, which are called 'tonification methods' (Brimhana). Reduction therapies include methods for increasing Agni, reducing Ama and decreasing the doshas of Vata, Pitta and Kapha. Tonification methods aim mainly at increasing the tissues but also aid in revitalization and rejuvenation (Rasayana), strengthen immunity and promote longevity.

Following this therapeutic model, many types of marma therapy have arisen that cover the entire range of natural treatment modalities including the use of massage, oils, herbs and various instruments like needles to stimulate marma points. Marma therapy can be employed as part of daily and seasonal life-style practices (Dinacharya, Ritucharya) or part of complex clinical procedures to eradicate the doshas (Pancha Karma). Besides treating the body, marma therapy can be used for pranic healing or energy medicine in various forms. It can also be used for calming the mind, calming the emotions and stress reduction. Marma therapy is a great aid for Yoga and meditation, facilitating the opening up of consciousness on an inner level.

Marma therapy is usually supplementary to other Ayurvedic therapies, whether constitutional or disease focused, applied along with them for added enhancement. We have already examined in the previous chapter the yogic methods of marma therapy. Here we will examine the medical methods. We can identify ten main medical methods of treating marmas, which can be divided into three groups.

Methods of Marma Therapy

I. Massage and Energy Methods

1. Abhyanga or Massage—Using various forms of pressure and movement with the hands or other parts of the body like the feet and elbows. This is aided by applying heavy oils like sesame or special Ayurvedic medicated herbal oils (tailas), so it includes not only massage but also oil therapy. Some forms of Ayurvedic massage may use dry powders, so many techniques fall under it.

2. Aroma Therapy—Using aromatic oils like sandalwood or camphor on marmas. This may be combined with massage or Abhyanga.

3. Mardana or Acupressure—Strong application of pressure on particular marmas, which may be combined with the use of special massage oils or aromatic oils done as part of massage.

4. Pranic or Energy Healing—Directing Prana either at a distance or through therapeutic touch, not requiring but often enhanced by the use of massage techniques and oils.

II. Herbal Methods

5. Lepa or Applying Herbal Pastes—Use of herbal pastes like sandalwood, turmeric and ginger or various herbal ointments on different marmas.

6. Herbal Treatment—Taking herbs internally in the form of pills and decoctions as well as applying them externally to marmas in the form of poultices (which overlaps with the use of herbal pastes).

III. Use of Instruments

7. Sira Vedha (Vessel Piercing) and Blood-letting—Piercing (vedha) of veins or vessels (sira), particularly blood-letting or bleeding of marma points.

8. Suchi-karma or Acupuncture—Piercing (vedha) with needles (suchi) or acupuncture, including puncturing of small vessels at marma points.

9. Agni-karma or Heat Application—Methods of heat (Agni) application (karma) to marma regions, including the use of heated rods and moxibustion.

10. Ksharakarma or Cautery—Application (karma) of herbal alkalis (ksharas) or caustic substances near marma points like chemical cautery.

The first group of four methods—massage, aroma therapy, acupressure and pranic healing—are usually used together. They generally require a therapist but can be done on a limited scope as a form of self-treatment. The second group of herbal methods can be used along with massage methods or by themselves. They require a working knowledge of herbs to utilize. The third group of four methods employs various instruments like magnets, rods, needles or caustic substances. These are generally strong in nature and require a good clinical knowledge for their application.

We will discuss the first two groups of methods—the massage and herbal methods in the current chapter. The third group, which is more technical in nature, is described briefly in the Appendix for reference purposes (Part III, 1. Use of Instruments to Treat Marmas: Blood-letting, Acupuncture, Agni-karma and Kshara-karma, Part III, 2. Marmapuncture, Ayurvedic Acupuncture).

I. Massage and Energy Methods of Marma Therapy

Therapeutic touch is the main method for treating marmas, just as it is the main method for treating the surface of the body where most marmas are located. In yogic philosophy, touch is the sensory power that corresponds to the cosmic air element. The air element in turn relates to Prana or the cosmic life-force. Touch conveys Prana, which is the main healing power of life. The Prana from the practitioner affects the marma, which itself is a pranic center where our vital energy easily gets impaired. Prana at a deeper level carries the energy of love and consciousness, so therapeutic touch can help heal the mind and heart as well as the body.

Good Ayurvedic doctors develop a strong power of Prana, both from their medical practice and from their yogic practices (particularly Pranayama), which is an integral part of an Ayurvedic life-style. A highly evolved Ayurvedic doctor can heal marma points by his pranic power alone. We must not overlook this healing power of the therapist. *A practitioner with good Prana can achieve good results even without a great deal of technical skill or much time spent in treating a marma point.* On the other hand, a practitioner with little development of Prana may not be very effective, even if technically correct in their treatment.

1. Marma Massage/ Oil Massage

Abhyanga or massage is the main Ayurvedic method of treating marmas. It employs not only massage techniques but also the use of special massage oils, to which special herbs and aromas may be added to extend the healing energy to all regions of the body. Abhyanga combines the power of therapeutic touch along with the medicinal properties of oils, herbs and aromas.

For the strongest treatment level, massage of specific marmas is conducted along with whole body massage as an added enhancement. Whole body massage opens marma energy in general and makes individual marmas more accessible for treatment. Another method consists of 're-gional massage'—first massaging the area of the body where the marma is located. This means that a facial or head massage can be given before treating marmas on the head. Similarly, massages of the arms and hands, legs and feet, or back or front of the body can be given before treating the marmas located in those areas. Such regional massage helps open the energy in that part of the body and makes specific marma massage more effective. It is also not as time-consuming as whole body massage. However, individual marmas can be massaged by themselves without any additional massage as a limited or quick form of treatment.

The different methods of Ayurvedic massage are prescribed according to season, environmental conditions, disease condition and individual constitution. We will define them here mainly according to doshic constitution.

Marma Massage

Marmas are sensitive areas, so massage should be done carefully, using mainly the thumb, which projects the main pranic power of the hand. However, the knuckle, wrist, palm of the hand or heel of the foot can be used in certain conditions, particularly to cover larger regions. The duration of massage for marma points should be at least three to five minutes twice a day. For massage two important rules should be remembered.

1. Perform the massage motion in a *clockwise* motion when tonification or strengthening the internal organs and tissues is the aim.

Imagine putting a clock on the body of the patient and then follow the movement of the clock's hand forward from right to left as it progresses from 12 to 1, 2, 3 and so on.

2. Perform the massage in a *counterclockwise* manner when the goal is to

reduce excess doshas or excess tissues growth or for detoxification purposes.

Imagine putting clock on the body of the patient and then follow the movement of the clock's hand backward from left to right to left from 12 to 11, 10, 9 and so on.

Oils for Marma Massage

Massage often requires the use of heavy or fatty oils like sesame or almond. Their oily or emollient quality softens the skin and reduces friction, making the massage more pleasant. Such oils can penetrate into marmas, loosen tension, relieve pain and bring nourishment to the skin and muscles in the region.

Ayurvedic oil therapy or *Snehana* employs different oils in various contexts to either strengthen the patient or remove toxins, depending upon the nature of the oil and the amount used.

- Most heavy oils like sesame or almond are heating in nature and are generally used for Vata, which benefits from using them in large amounts.
- Some oils are light and spicy and good for Kapha, like mustard or safflower. Heavier oils that are heating in nature, even sesame, can also be used for Kapha but the amount applied should be small.
- Only a few oils are cooling in nature and are better for Pitta. Such are coconut, ghee (clarified butter) and sunflower oil.
- However, we should note that such heavy oils are not used, or used only sparingly, in cases of Ama (toxins in the digestive tract evidenced by thick tongue coating), when there is a cold, flu or fever, or in other acute conditions. Heavy oils can suppress Agni (the digestive fire) and help hold toxins and pathogens in the body.

Massage Oils and Doshic Indications

Dosha	Main Massage Oils
Vata	Sesame, almond, olive, ghee
Pitta	Coconut, sunflower, safflower, ghee
Kapha	Mustard, safflower, apricot, sesame (small amounts)

Special Ayurvedic Medicated Oils (Tailas)

Ayurveda uses various medicated oils called 'tailas' from 'tila' meaning sesame oil, which is the main oil base these are made with. Tailas consist of fatty oils like sesame or coconut in which various herbs are cooked, some of which like sandalwood or camphor may be aromatic. This allows the properties of herbs to enter into the oil and add their effects. Herbs used include tonics like ashwagandha, bala and shatavari and nervines like brahmi and gotu kola. Tailas are usually named after the main herbs in them like Ashwagandha Taila, a sesame oil preparation dominated by the herb ashwagandha. They offer a greater herbal effect to the use of massage oils. *Tailas are often the best way to treat marmas because they combine massage oils and herbs for a more powerful synergistic action.* Not all of them have pleasant aromatic properties, however.

A number of Ayurvedic massage oils are mentioned relative to the treatment of marmas. These Tailas are listed in the *Appendix 5*. Many of these are now available from Ayurvedic stores and companies in the United States.

2. Aroma Therapy

Aromatic oils have powerful effects upon marmas, serving to radiate their influence to the different channels, organs and systems of the body and mind. Aromas can penetrate deep into marmas and adjust their energy level and frequency. They can reduce excess doshas or bring in subtle healing energies of Prana (primary vitality), Tejas (primary radiance) and Ojas (immune power). Aroma therapy for marma points is both one of the most powerful forms of aroma therapy as well as one of the best forms of marma therapy.

Aroma therapy is a quick and easy method of working on marmas that can be applied either by itself or as part of massage. Generally, it is stronger if it is combined with massage of the point. One can apply an aromatic oil before massage in order to open the energy of the point. Or one can anoint the marma with an aromatic oil once a massage is over in order to help complete and seal the treatment.

Applying an aromatic oil as a treatment in itself, one can anoint a marma point as a kind of quick or instant treatment. This is particularly good for acute conditions or if one does not have the time for a fuller treatment. Use cooling and sedating oils like sandalwood to relieve pain, inflammation or irritation at the site. Use warming and stimulating oils like cinnamon or eucalyptus to remove cold and stiffness or to promote circulation in the region. Various pain balms like Tiger balm, which contain mainly camphor, menthol or wintergreen can be used this way as well.

Generally, it is best to work an aromatic oil into a marma region using one's fingers or thumb, even if little other massage will be done. Just as in the case of marma massage, use a clockwise motion of massage to strengthen the energy at a marma and a counterclockwise motion to reduce it.

Some aromatic oils like sandalwood can be used instead of heavy oils like sesame for general massage purposes as well. Hot-natured aromatic oils like eucalyptus can be used like rubbing alcohol or prepared in rubbing alcohol as penetrating massage agents.

You may wish to wash off any excess aromatic oils if you don't want a lingering fragrance (though this is often helpful therapeutically). Or, you can apply aromatic oils to marmas before sleep and then shower the oil off in the morning.

Types of Aromatic Oils

Aromatic oils are of several major types. Most common are 'spicy' or pungent aromatic oils. These are usually heating in nature and good for reducing Kapha and Vata. Typical spicy oils include anise, basil, bay, calamus, eucalyptus, ginger, heena, nutmeg, pepper, sage and thyme. Most oils that derive from coniferous trees are of this type as well, such as cedar, Himalayan cedar, fir, juniper, pine and spruce.

Some spicy oils are more aromatic than heating and can be used to some degree for all three doshic types, with fewer restrictions on Pitta than other spicy oils. Such oils include camphor, cardamom, cinnamon, cloves, coriander, cumin, fennel, mint, motherwort, rosemary, saffron, spearmint, turmeric and wintergreen.

Another important type of aromatic oils is 'sweet oils', which are generally derived from flowers. These are good for reducing Pitta and Vata but can increase Kapha. They are effective for gynecological complaints and are tonics to the heart and the reproductive system. Such fragrances are champak, evening primrose, frangipani, gardenia, honeysuckle, iris, jasmine, lily, lotus, rose and saffron.

Certain oils derived from tree resins have special healing properties for treating injuries, musculo-skeletal pain, stiffness and arthritis. These are often good for all three doshas and are particularly useful for Vata and Kapha. Such are frankincense, guggul, myrrh and shallaki, as well as the resins of various conifers (particularly pines).

A few oils are earthy and slightly sulfury in smell. These are particularly good for Vata and for stabilizing of consciousness in conditions of shock or hysteria. Such are garlic, onion, valerian, jatamamsi and asafoetida (hing).

Aromatic Oils and Doshic Indications

The following are generally good aromatic oils for the different doshas. Note that many fragrances can help reduce all three doshas. The doshic application of aromas is not as strict as that of foods or herbs.

Just as Ayurvedic herbalism employs many diverse herbal formulas and compounds, formulas combining several aromatic oils can also be devised. Ayurvedic practitioners often devise their own aromatic blends, just as they do various herbal combinations. The general rule is that several herbs or oils in a formula will have a stronger therapeutic effect than the same amount of any single herb or oil. This is owing to the synergistic effect that occurs from combining related healing substances. Special Ayurvedic aroma combinations have been developed for treating various marmas.

Aromatic Oils, Spices and Flower Essences	
Vata	Ajwan, almond, aloes wood (agaru), angelica, anise, asafoetida (hing), basil (tulsi), bay leaves, birch, black pepper, cajeput, calamus, camphor, caraway, cardamom, cayenne, cedar, cinnamon, cloves, cumin, eucalyptus, fennel, frangipani, frankincense, garlic, gardenia, geranium, ginger, guggul, heena, jasmine, jatamamsi, lavender, lemon, licorice, lotus, musk (floral), myrrh, nutmeg, orange, rose, sage, turmeric, valerian, vanilla, wintergreen
Pitta	Camphor, cardamom, chamomile, champak, chrysanthemum, cloves, coriander, evening primrose, fennel, gardenia, geranium, honeysuckle, iris, jasmine, jatamamsi, khus, lemongrass, licorice, lily, lime, lotus, mint, myrrh, rose, saffron, sandalwood, turmeric, vanilla, wintergreen, wormwood, yarrow
Kapha	Ajwan, anise, artemesia, angelica, asafoetida (hing), basil (tulsi), bay leaves, bayberry, birch, black pepper, cajeput, calamus, camphor, caraway, cardamom, cayenne, cedar, cloves, cinnamon, elecampane, eucalyptus, frangipani, frankincense, fir, garlic, ginger, guggul, heena, hyssop, juniper, lemon, marjoram, mugwort, musk (floral), mustard, myrrh, nutmeg, parsley, pennyroyal, peppermint, pine, pippali, rosemary, rue, sage, spruce, tea tree, thyme, turmeric, valerian, wintergreen, wormwood

Combination of Heavy Oils and Aromatic Oils

Different oils and aromas have specific therapeutic effects that can greatly enhance the efficacy of massage. For balancing the doshas, the following oils can be used on different marmas.[1]

VATA TYPE INDIVIDUALS OR CONDITIONS OF HIGH VATA (deficient tissues, tremors, pain or insomnia):

This requires the use of heavy or fatty oils like sesame, almond or castor oil. Warm aromatic oils like ginger and cinnamon or calming oils like sandalwood or rose are also good, but *generally Vatas require a liberal application of heavier oils like sesame to really ground them.* Some high Vata types may be sensitive or disturbed by any strong fragrances, even those which are usually good for their type.

PITTA TYPE INDIVIDUALS OR CONDITIONS OF HIGH PITTA (excess heat, fever, bleeding or anger):

This requires cooling massage oils like coconut, sunflower or ghee along with sweet and cooling fragrances like sandalwood, rose or khus (vetiver), or along with aromatic oils that reduce Pitta but improve digestion like cloves or coriander. *Often the use of sweet aromatic oils is enough to bring down high Pitta conditions like fever or irritability, particularly the use of sandalwood.*

However, many Pitta men who could benefit from the use of sweet fragrances may be unwilling to use them because of the feminine connotations of the fragrance. If this is the case, one can use sandalwood, khus, cloves or mint, which reduce Pitta without leaving a strong flowery aroma like rose or jasmine.

FOR KAPHA TYPE INDIVIDUALS OR CONDITIONS OF HIGH KAPHA (excess tissues, fluids or mucus):

This requires lighter application of warming massage oils like mustard along with hot and penetrating aromas like eucalyptus, cinnamon or mint. *Often the use of hot aromatic oils or pastes of spicy herbs like eucalyptus, camphor, ginger or calamus is enough to reduce Kapha conditions of congestion or dullness.* Kapha types like sweet and flowery fragrances but these are not good for them.

How Oil Massage and Aroma Therapy Compare

Ayurvedic massage is part of oleation (Snehana) therapy. Oleation is part of detoxification or reduction therapy (Shodhana) used for loosening toxins in the bones, joints, muscles and skin. The use of hot aromatic oils or herbs is part of sweating or sudation (Swedana) therapy, which is also part of this same type of therapy. It aims at drawing toxins out through the blood and skin. In Ayurveda, oleation and sweating therapies (Snehana and Swedana) are used together to help draw the doshas out of the deeper tissues and bring them through the circulatory system and into the digestive tract for their elimination from the body by other therapeutic methods (note the theory of Pancha Karma as explained in various books on Ayurveda).[2]

This means that oil massage and aroma therapy on marma points can be viewed as a special or localized Snehana-Swedana therapy. It can be practiced along with Pancha Karma. It is very effective for points on the head and problems of headache and sinusitis. Oil massage and aroma therapy to marmas on the head helps remove toxins from the region of Prana and harmonizes the movement of Prana in the mind and the nervous system.

The use of heavy oils like sesame or almond is also part of Ayurvedic tonification (Brimhana) therapy and is indicated for conditions of low body weight, poor tissue development and high Vata. For tonification purposes, it is important to combine oil application to selected marmas with whole body massage, using large quantities of oil. Oil drips to various marma regions, particularly the forehead (shirodhara), can be helpful as well. Oil enemas (combining half a cup of sesame oil and half a cup of warm water) are even more powerful as they work on Vata's site of accumulation in the colon.

On the other hand, the use of hot spices and aromatic oils is part of reduction therapy (Langhana), indicated mainly for conditions of excess body weight, high Kapha and Ama (accumulated toxins). It is part of Ayurvedic palliation (Shamana) therapy, which aims at increasing the digestive power or Agni in order to burn up toxins (Ama). The use of hot aromatic oils on certain marma regions is good for weight reduction, stimulating digestion and promoting detoxification.

Oils and aromas can be used to manage different types of pain. Heavy oils like sesame or almond are better for pain owing to weakness or stiffness (Vata). Hot aromatic oils like ginger or eucalyptus are better for pain owing to cold or congestion (Kapha). Cool aromatic oils like sandalwood or khus (vetiver) are better for pain owing to inflammation (Pitta).

3. Mardana (Acupressure)

Mardana is another method of Ayurvedic massage meaning 'applying pressure'. We can also call it 'acupressure'. Mardana is particularly suitable for usage on marmas, especially smaller points of one finger unit or less in size (the majority of marmas), where the bodily energy is concentrated.

Acupressure consists of applying pressure to the marma, using the thumb or fingers, particularly the index or middle fingers, which can hold a greater force. It is particularly good for marmas on the extremities (legs and arms) or on the head, which are of easy access. Acupressure can be done on sore or sensitive points (unless injured) until the pain and tension is released. One can use the thumb or the nail of the thumb for a more pointed pressure. This works well if combined along with the index finger for marmas like Kurcha that one can grasp from both sides. In larger and deeper-seated marmas, like those on the hips or back, the elbow can be used for greater pressure when necessary.

Method of Ayurvedic Acupressure
- Locate the respective marma region and apply a steady and moderate pressure with the thumb or finger, starting slowly and gently and gradually increasing in strength.

- Just as with marma massage, use a slight circular motion *clockwise in direction* when tonification or strengthening the internal organs and tissues is the aim.
- When the goal is to reduce excess doshas or excess tissues, apply a slight circular motion in a *counterclockwise* manner.
- Continue to apply pressure for three to five minutes or until the patient feels relief.
- Lightly massage the area to disperse any tension.

Ayurvedic acupressure is best done as part of overall body massage. It also works better, particularly on Vata types, if done with massage oils like sesame. It is good to end acupressure treatment with the application of aromatic oils to aid in restoring circulation into the area.

The use of aromatic oils with acupressure is similar to that relative to marma massage, so most of what was said there applies here as well. While more complex massage oils and aromas can be used as per the indications of the marma, the following simple recommendations can be followed in most instances:

- For Vata, plain sesame or almond oils are good to use along with acupressure. For aromatic oils, cinnamon or calamus are best.
- For Pitta, sandalwood oil is the best general oil/aroma. Clove oil can be used when the intention is more to stimulate the point.
- For Kapha, it is best to use stimulating aromatic oils like camphor, cinnamon or eucalyptus along with acupressure.

The Five Pranas

The five Pranas relate to the five fingers. We can use different fingers to project the different types of Prana to various marma points.

- Prana relates to the thumb.
- Udana relates to the index finger.
- Vyana relates to the middle finger.
- Samana relates to the ring finger.
- Apana relates to the little finger.
- The palm carries the energy of all five Pranas and of Prana itself.

The five Pranas have their different roles in massage. Prana itself affords us overall energy. Udana allows our energy to move upward and holds the body erect. Apana moves downward and reflects the force of gravity, giving stability and grounding us. Vyana moves outward, expanding and releasing, while Samana moves inward, holding and conserving.

This means that we can use the force of Prana to energize marmas, that of Udana to stimulate them, that of Apana to ground them, that of Vyana to expand and release their energy, and that of Samana to contract and hold their energy. This can be done by the type of massage performed, by the type of oils used or by how the therapist directs his or her Prana during the treatment. A simple way to do this is relative to which fingers we use for acupressure.

Acupressure done with the thumb strengthens Prana overall. Acupressure done with the index finger projects the upward moving energy of Udana. That done with the middle finger projects the outward moving energy of Vyana. That done with the ring finger projects the contracting and consolidating energy of Samana. That done with the little finger projects the downward moving energy of Apana. However, an Ayurvedic practitioner must have a good pranic energy in order to do this.

In addition we can massage the fingers of the hands and the toes of the foot in order to work on these different types of Prana that they hold. This is a kind of special Ayurvedic hand and foot massage.

4. Pranic or Energy Healing

Pranic or Energy Healing, called *Prana Chikitsa* in Sanskrit, is an integral part of Ayurvedic massage. Much of what we have already said relative to massage applies to it as well, but it can also be done by itself. In this practice one simply uses ones Prana on the marma point. In large marma zones like the heart or the navel, one can simply put the palm of the hands on top of the marma, or a small distance of a few inches above it in order to bring in positive pranic energy and disperse negative energy. Another method is to touch the marma and use the pressure of the touch (including acupressure) to convey Prana to the client.

In pranic healing, where one aims at the transmission of energy from the healer to the client, the massage technique may be of little importance. For this the Prana of the healer is the main focus. In pranic treatments, it is best to direct Prana along with your breath, projecting positive vitality along with your inhalation and removing negative energy along with your exhalation. pranic healing combines well with other yogic methods mentioned in the last chapter like Pratyahara and mantra, including the use of colors and gems. It also goes well with Polarity Therapy,[3] which itself is a kind of pranic healing. Another method that can be used along with pranic healing is the use of magnets or magnet therapy. And, of course, when one is performing massage, one should always consider the positive flow of Prana to the client.

---

[1] Note *Ayurveda and Aroma Therapy* (Light and Brian Miller).

[2] Note *Ayurveda and Panchakarma* (Joshi).

[3] Note *The Ayurvedic Guide to Polarity Therapy* (Morningstar).

CHAPTER 6

The Many Methods of Marma Therapy 2: Herbal Methods

Herbs, which convey the pranic force of nature, are the main medicines used in Ayurvedic treatment. Ayurveda uses herbs 'energetically' according to their taste (rasa), heating capacity (virya), post-digestive effect (vipaka) and other such factors.[1] This allows herbs to target specific doshas, tissues and systems in order to counter disease and increase positive vitality. There are special herbs for treating all the systems of the body and all diseases.

Herbs have their special usage in marma therapy. They can be applied externally on the marma for direct treatment. Herbs can also be taken internally to aid in healing at the marma site. In this way, a broad range of herbal therapies can be used as part of marma therapy. A complete marma therapy should always include the taking of herbs.

1. Marma Therapy with Herbal Pastes

Treatment by applying herbal pastes is called *Lepa Chikitsa* or 'paste therapy'. It is much like the western herbal usage of poultices, except in Ayurveda generally an oil like sesame is added to powdered herbs in order to make a paste. The oil allows the herbs to adhere better as well as helping the herbal properties penetrate through the skin. Demulcent herbs like aloe gel can be used instead of oil, as can honey in some instances.

Herbal pastes help reduce swelling and pain when applied over an injured marma. They afford strength and stability to injured bones and joints. Pastes are sometimes applied after massage in order to seal the energy of the treatment and continue its healing effects. There are three types of *Lepa* according to the thickness of the herbal paste:

1. *Pralepa*—Thin paste
2. *Pradeha*—Thick paste
3. *Alepa*—Medium paste

Alepa or a medium paste is used more often. To create this, get a suitable quantity of the powder of the herb to be used (generally one or two ounces). Then add oil or ghee ¼ part to the amount of the herb for treating Vata conditions, 1/6 part for Pitta and 1/8 part for Kapha. Use sufficient oil to create a consistent paste that will adhere to the skin. Then apply the paste over the marma. Apply the paste opposite to the direction of the bodily hair. Then it is less likely to irritate the skin.

Ghee is the best oil to use for cooling and anti-inflammatory actions, including treatment for burns and sunburns and for most Pitta conditions. Sesame oil is best for pain relief, for countering dryness and protecting the bones and joints and for most Vata and Kapha conditions. Castor oil is good with herbs for treating injuries and swelling.

- Herbal pastes of spicy herbs like ginger, calamus, nutmeg, bayberry or cloves can be applied for headache, nasal congestion or sinusitis at marmas on the head like Sthapani, Shankha or Phana marmas. The combination of ginger, calamus and cloves is excellent for such purposes.

- Herbal pastes of carminative (gas-dispelling) herbs to Nabhi marma (navel) are excellent for countering cramping, bloating and distention. Asafoetida (hing) is good for this purpose.

- Turmeric paste is good for minor injuries and for improving circulation to marmas for all the doshas. However, it does leave a yellowish stain on clothes or skin.

- Sandalwood paste is good for cooling and stress-relieving action, reduction of Pitta and Vata, and calming the mind and heart. It can be used on many marmas for this purpose much like sandalwood oil.

- Aloe gel is great for cooling action on marmas, relieving inflammation, irritation or sunburn at the affected area. It can be combined with powdered herbs like turmeric or sandalwood in order to strengthen its cooling and healing action.

- For soft tissue injuries, pastes of herbs like turmeric and aloe gel, or poultices of green herbs like comfrey leaf or plantain are helpful.

- For injuries to the joints or bones, use pastes of bone tonic herbs like comfrey root, ashwagandha, nirgundi or Siberian ginseng that promote healing and strengthen the bone tissue.

- Honey is a good ingredient for herbal pastes in the case of burns or wounds. It has a natural antiseptic action.

- Ghee (clarified butter) is also excellent for burns, rashes and inflammations.

2. Herbal Treatment of Marmas

Ayurveda uses different herbal teas, powders and pills, including a number of special formulas and preparations as part of its vast pharmaceutical industry. As marmas relate to key vital points on the body and important vital organs, many herbs can be used in their treatment. For treating marmas, external application of herbs to the specific marma often goes along with ingestion of the herbs in order to treat the body as a whole.

Note that the herbs and dosages recommended for internal usage are only general. Please consult an herbal text for more precise information before taking such herbs.[2]

Two great herbs for overall treatment of marmas are *turmeric* and *guggul*. Turmeric is excellent for all soft tissue injury, for improving healing at marma points and increasing circulation to marma regions. Guggul is perhaps the best overall herb for marma therapy, working well on both soft tissue and bone injuries, relieving pain and restoring energy flow. It is excellent for keeping marma points free of obstruction or blockages.

1. Treatment for Pain

Charaka indicated using special pain-relieving or analgesic herbs (the Vedana-sthapana group of herbs) for pain relief at different marmas.[3] Many herbs of a strongly spicy or bitter taste and aromatic nature have this property.

- Important herbs in the pain-relieving group include bayberry, cloves, guggul, tulsi (basil), shallaki, prasarini, nirgundi, jatamamsi, kadamba, mocharas, willow, padmaka (wild cherry), Himalayan cedar (devadaru) and shala.
- Additional western herbs of similar properties are wintergreen, valerian, lady's slipper, kava kava, chaparral, birch, licorice and myrrh. The Chinese herb corydalis is also very good.
- Ayurvedic formulas like *Yogaraj Guggul* (for joint pain) and *Mahayogaraj Guggul* (for nerve pain) are great, if available.

Such herbs are generally taken internally in dosages of 1 - 3 grams three times a day in the form of powders or herbal teas for short term usage, but please note their specific indications in various herb books. They can also be applied in the form of a paste on the marma to be treated. Some are also available in ointment form like Tiger balm, Ayurvedic pain balms and ointments using wintergreen, mint, camphor or other pain-relieving and muscle-relaxant herbs.

2. Treatment for Bleeding

Sushruta as a surgeon indicated various methods for controlling bleeding including ligation of bleeding vessels, cautery, pressure bandages, cold water or ice and the use of certain hemostatic or 'stopping-bleeding' herbs.[4] Many such herbs can be found in nature.

- Ayurvedic herbs in this stopping-bleeding group consist mainly of astringents like turmeric, sandalwood, alum, lotus, nagakeshara, barks of pancha valkala (five fig trees), durva, laksha, gojihva and padmaka. The mineral alum, which is a strong astringent, is also excellent.
- Additional western herbs include arnica, plantain, yarrow, comfrey, mullein, white oak bark, aloe and alum root. Also excellent is the Chinese patent medicine Yunnan Bai Yao.

Such herbs are generally taken internally in dosages of 1 - 3 grams three times a day in the form of powders or herbal teas for short term usage, but please note their specific indications in various herb books. They can be applied in the form of a paste or poultice on the marma to be treated.

3. Swelling and Edema

To relieve swelling and edema at the site of injury, Sushruta suggests several different water-dispelling herbs.

- Ayurvedic herbs for this include stimulants and diuretics like turmeric, ginger, tulsi, nirgundi, gokshura, Himalayan cedar, mocharas and shilajit, as well as leaves of lemon and onion.
- Turmeric paste is good by itself and can be mixed with dry ginger powder to promote circulation to the region.
- Many diuretic herbs can be used internally like juniper berries, cubebs, plantain, uva ursi, coriander or lemongrass.
- Pastes of certain tree resins like myrrh, guggul, fir or pine can be applied to the marma for this purpose.

Such herbs are generally taken internally in dosages of 1 - 3 grams three times a day in the form of powders or herbal teas for short term usage. Again please note their specific indications in various herb books. They can be applied in the form of a paste or poultice on the marma to be treated.

4. To Counter Shock

Charaka suggests using the Consciousness-holding (Samjna-sthapana) group of herbs for revival from shock.[5] Such herbs are generally spicy and aromatic in nature. They open the mind and senses and allow the Prana to move throughout the nervous system.

- Such conscious-reviving herbs are asafoetida (hing), bayberry, calamus, tulsi, garlic, camphor, musk, bayberry, guduchi, jatamamsi, valerian, shankhapushpi, guggul, brahmi (gotu kola) and ashoka, most of which have strong odors as aromatic oils.
- For quickly reviving a person, have them inhale a snuff of hing (asafoetida), calamus or ginger powder. Hing is best and will bring down Vata as well.
- Another method is to crush a clove of garlic and put some of the juice at the base of the nostrils and in the mouth of the person. Or have the person inhale a penetrating aromatic oil like camphor, eucalyptus or menthol.
- Ayurveda has special eye creams (collyriums or anjanas) to apply around the eyes. These are also very helpful.
- If shock is owing to cold or poor circulation, use warming stimulants like cayenne, ginger or mustard taken in the mouth.
- Once the patient is awake, have them drink warming and stimulating herbal teas like ginger, cinnamon or cardamom to stimulate their circulation.

Once the patient is revived, give them a warm bath with a little ghee, sesame oil, milk or coconut juice added to the bath water. This restores the bodily fluids. Administer a cool sponge bath using a little sandalwood oil or powder when shock has occurred owing to heat or fever.

Such herbs are sometimes taken internally in the form of powders or herbal teas for short term usage. Some of these are powerful herbs like camphor that should not be taken internally except in very small amounts. Please note their specific indications in various herb books before using them. They can be applied in the form of a paste or poultice on the marma to be treated.

5. To Prevent Pus Formation on a Wound

Many common alterative or blood-cleansing herbs are good for preventing infection and promoting healing. These are usually bitter or astringent in taste. Of course, one must be careful if there is a high fever or severe infection.

- Externally, use herbs like aloe gel, turmeric, myrrh, comfrey, dandelion, plantain and yellow dock as pastes or poultices.

- Internally, use anti-bacterial herbs like golden seal, barberry, turmeric and katuka as powders or herbal teas.

Such herbs are generally taken internally in dosages of 1 - 3 grams three times a day in the form of powders or herbal teas for short term usage. But please note their specific indications in various herbals. They can be applied in the form of a paste or poultice on the marma to be treated.

The Ayurvedic text *Sahasrayoga* gives two excellent herbal formulas for healing of marmas that can be taken in pill form—*Brihat Marma Gutika* and *Laghu Marma Gutika*. Note *Appendix 5* for their ingredients.

6. Healing Wounds at Marmas

For healing wounds to marmas, there are many herbal combinations that can be used both internally and applied externally to the site as pastes or poultices.

- Turmeric or aloe gel can be used separately or mixed together. Many western herbs can be used the same way like comfrey, arnica and plantain, much like the herbs mentioned above for stopping-bleeding. This is mainly for external application, but taking small amounts of the herbs internally can also be helpful.
- For injuries affecting the bones or joints herbs like myrrh, arjuna, nirgundi, guggul, kava kava or Siberian ginseng are good, both internally and externally.
- For soft tissue damage and clearing out any stagnant blood, circulatory stimulants like turmeric, saffron, angelica, rose and manjishta (madder) are indicated. This is mainly for internal usage.

Honey applied externally is a simple and effective remedy to promote healing and stop infection. Ghee and butter are also good for external application in the case of burns and inflammation. To prevent scarring, the long-term use of an oil like sesame or vitamin E oil is good, applied daily until the wound is healed.

For internal usage of the herbs mentioned above, again generally follow the dosage of 1 - 3 grams three times a day in the form of powders or herbal teas for short-term usage Please note their specific indications in various herbals for more specific indications and for more long-term usage.

Two additional special Ayurvedic decoctions for injuries to marmas are *Marma Kashaya* and *Dhanvantara Kashaya*. These are mainly for internal usage. Note *Appendix 5* for their ingredients.

7. To Restore Vital Energy

If there has been severe injury to marmas, it is important that the patient undergo a long-term tonification and rejuvenation treatment to increase vitality (Ojas) and rebuild damaged tissues. For this purpose there are many special tonic herbs that can be used, like ashwagandha and ginseng. Such treatment, however, should be started only after the acute injury has healed. It may be continued for a long period of time, up to three to six months, when there is physical or nervous debility or exhaustion.

- For rebuilding the bones and muscles use tonic herbs like ashwagandha, bala, shilajit, astragalus, and ginseng.
- For restoring the blood and bodily fluids use tonic herbs like shatavari, marshmallow, American ginseng, rehmannia, and amalaki, or the Ayurvedic jelly 'Chyavan Prash'.
- For healing the nervous system, use nervine tonics like brahmi, gotu kola, shankhapushpi, jatamamsi, haritaki, and licorice.

Such herbs are generally taken internally in dosages of 1 - 3 grams three times a day in the form of powders or herbal teas and can generally be used for periods of one month or more. They are also good taken as milk decoctions (cooked in milk) or taken with ghee. They are usually combined with adequate rest, nutritive (tissue-rebuilding) diets, deep breathing exercises and restorative Yoga poses.

---

[1] Please examine books on Ayurveda like the *Yoga of Herbs* for information on the Ayurvedic view of herbs and their usage.

[2] Note books like the *Yoga of Herbs* (Frawley and Lad) and *Planetary Herbology* (Tierra).

[3] *Charaka Samhita Sutrasthana IV.47.*

[4] Sushruta Samhita Sutrasthana XIV.36.

[5] Charaka Samhita Sutrasthana IV.48.

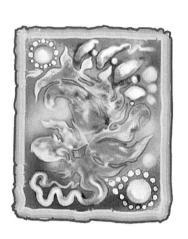

Part Two

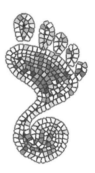

Table of Marmas and Their Treatment

The following section consists of a
table of the main 107 marmas,
delineating each marma
as well as its treatment.

CHAPTER 7

Overview of Table of Marmas and Marma Therapies

This section explains how to use the following Table of Marmas. Its emphasis is on preparing the reader to effectively use the therapies indicated under each marma. It also contains tables and illustrations correlating the marmas according to the doshas, subdoshas and channel-systems to aid in broader Ayurvedic treatment strategies. We recommend going over it carefully before proceeding to the individual marma descriptions.

The Table of Marmas describes each marma according to the Ayurvedic factors discussed in the first section of the book, as well as anatomically in modern medical terms. For those unfamiliar with Ayurvedic terms such as the doshas, subdoshas and srotamsi, please refer to the earlier chapters in which these are explained. For the anatomical terminology consult a medical dictionary if needed.

I. Overview of Marma Therapies

The Table of Marmas describes special treatments for each marma point described. *The following overview of treatment outlines simple methods for treating all marmas.* Its purpose is to enable the reader to treat any marma on a general level, even if he or she may lack the specific knowledge of oils and herbs necessary for detailed treatment. Please examine previous chapters for the details of marma therapy as needed. In addition, remember to treat the person as a whole. Marma therapy is an important adjunct to be applied along with other Ayurvedic therapies, diet and life-style modifications. It is usually given by those skilled in the broader field of Ayurveda.

However, marmas can be used for self-treatment as well. Many marma points, particularly those on the extremities of the body, are easy to reach for self-treatment with massage, acupressure, massage oils or aromatic oils. You can do this on a daily or weekly basis to aid in energy circulation or to counter chronic ailments. You can use specific marmas to treat headaches, digestive problems, insomnia and many other conditions that you may be suffering from. This kind of treatment is particularly good before taking showers or baths, which can follow in order to wash off any excess oil. However, it cannot substitute for treatment by another, which brings in a different and potentially transformative pranic source.

Massage, aroma therapy and acupressure are combined together under one treatment section for each marma. This is because massage oils and aromatic oils are usually used along with massage or acupressure.

1. Oil Massage

Oil application is usually the best treatment for conditions of high Vata or for debility conditions generally. Remember to apply oils warm, particularly for Vata. However, in cases of high Kapha, overweight or edema, it is not always necessary to use a massage oil. In these cases, dry massage is usually better. For simple treatment by oil massage, marmas can be massaged with the following oils:

• Sesame or almond oil for Vata types or conditions
• Coconut or sunflower oil for Pitta types or conditions
• Mustard or sesame oil (smaller amounts) for Kapha types or conditions

Carry out the massage as explained in the section on **Marma Massage, Chapter 5 (p. 66).**

Key Symptoms of High Doshas at Marma Points

Vata   Cold and dry sensations in the area, sensitivity to wind or expo sure, cracking or roughness of the skin, severe or cutting pain

Pitta   Hot and damp sensations in the area, oiliness of the skin, bleed ing, redness, skin rash, hot or burning pain

Kapha   Cold and damp sensations in the area, paleness or whiteness of skin, swelling, fatty deposits, congestion, edema, dull ache

2. Aroma Therapy

The use of spicy, penetrating oils is specific for conditions of high Kapha or conditions of stagnation and congestion generally. The use of sweet fragrances is specific for conditions of high Pitta or conditions of fever and inflammation generally. For simple treatment by aroma therapy, marmas can be massaged or anointed with the following oils.

• A combination of spicy and sweet oils like ginger, cinnamon, sandalwood and rose is good for Vata.
• Cooling sweet oils like sandalwood, rose or lotus are good for Pitta.

• Spicy penetrating oils like eucalyptus, camphor or mint are best for Kapha.

Note that many of the specific treatments in terms of oils and herbs mentioned under different marmas can be used on other marmas when there are similar problems. Also note the formulas below.

Simple Marma Oils

ANTI-VATA OIL
Take ½ cup of sesame oil. Heat until slightly warm (not too hot or the aromatic oils will disperse) and add a few drops of sandalwood oil and calamus oil (if you cannot get calamus oil use cinnamon oil). Use the mixture slightly warm, but not so hot as to evaporate the aromatic oils.

ANTI-PITTA OIL
Take ½ cup of coconut oil and heat to slightly warm. Add several drops of sandalwood oil and a little rose oil, until a mild fragrance is produced. Then let the mixture cool for usage.

ANTI-KAPHA OIL
Take ¼ cup of sesame oil and ½ cup of mustard oil and mix together (using sesame and mustard oil in ratios of one to two), heating slightly. Add a few drops of camphor oil, menthol or wintergreen until a good fragrance is created.

3. Acupressure

Acupressure or finger pressure is specifically indicated for treating many different marmas. It is an important method for stimulating marma energy, particularly for smaller marmas or for trigger points within larger marmas. Generally a strong level of pressure with the thumb or middle finger can be used for Kapha, medium for Pitta, and more gentle for Vata, but be careful to note how painful each marma point may be and do not hurt the patient.

4. Pranic and Energy Healing

This can easily be done on any marma, using either the fingers or the palm of the hand. It depends upon the Prana of the healer, which should be strong and pure.

Other Treatment Methods

Additional treatment methods like acupuncture and heat application are mentioned for a few marmas by way of example. Such therapies can be used on most marmas, but may require more training in order to apply effectively. Please examine the *Appendix 1* and *Appendix 2* for more details on these therapies.

Yogic Methods

Yoga practices like meditation, mantra, Pratyahara and Pranayama have been mentioned for several important marmas, particularly relative to the chakras and nadis that they rule over. Holding the mind and Prana (our power of attention) at marmas aids in their healing and facilitates their energization at an internal level. We have not mentioned gems or colors much relative to specific marmas but their general application can be used here as well.

II. Marmas and the Doshas

Below are some prime correlations between the marmas, doshas, subdoshas and tissues of the body. This can help us understand how to use various marmas. These correlations are only by way of predominance. Most marmas can be used to treat any of the doshas depending upon the treatment methods and substances used.

1. Marmas and the Three Doshas

VATA	
Arms and Legs	Kshipra, Talahridaya*, Manibandha, Gulpha
Abdomen and Chest	Guda*, Basti, Nabhi, Apalapa
Hips and Back	Katikataruna, Amsa*, Amsaphalaka
Neck and Head	Adhipati*, Simanta, Sthapani, Vidhura, Krikatika, Shankha, Utkshepa, Avarta
PITTA	
Arms and Legs	Kurcha*, Kurchashira, Indrabasti, Kurpara (right), Janu (right)
Abdomen and Chest	Nabhi*, Hridaya, Apastambha
Hips and Back	Kukundara*, Brihati
Neck and Head	Nila, Sira Matrika, Apanga, Sthapani*, Adhipati
KAPHA	
Arms and Legs	Kshipra, Kurpara (left), Ani, Urvi*, Bahvi, Lohitaksha, Kakshadhara, Janu (left), Vitapa, Gulpha
Abdomen and Chest	Hridaya*, Stanamula, Stanarohita, Apastambha, Apalapa
Hips and Back	Nitamba*, Parshvasandhi, Brihati, Amsaphalaka
Neck and Head	Manya, Phana*, Shringataka

*These mark the most important marmas for the corresponding regions of the body.

2. Marma Points and the Subdoshas

The following are a few key connections between marma points and the subdoshas or five forms of Vata, Pitta and Kapha.

Vata Subtypes and Marma Points	
1. Prana Vayu	Adhipati and Sthapani marmas on the head relate to Prana Vayu and to the crown (Sahasrara) chakra. They control the mind and the central nervous system. Phana and Vidhura marmas are also good for Prana as circulation in the head and senses. Kshipra and Talahridaya are good for general stimulation of Prana and its entry into the body.
2. Udana Vayu	Nila, Manya, Krikatika and Amsa marmas on the neck and shoulders relate to Udana Vayu and to the throat chakra.
3. Vyana Vayu	Hridaya (heart), Brihati and Amsaphalaka marmas relate to Vyana Vayu and the heart chakra. Several marmas on the hands and feet are connected with Vyana as well as Prana, particularly Talahridaya and Kshipra.
4. Samana Vayu	Nabhi (navel), Apastambha and Kurchashira marmas relate to Samana Vayu and the navel chakra.
5. Apana Vayu	Basti (bladder), Guda (anus) and Vitapa (perineum) marmas relate to Apana Vayu and the two lower chakras. Marmas on the legs and feet like Talahridaya and Lohitaksha are connected to Apana as well as to Vyana. Utkshepa marma on the head has an overall control of Apana and Vata.

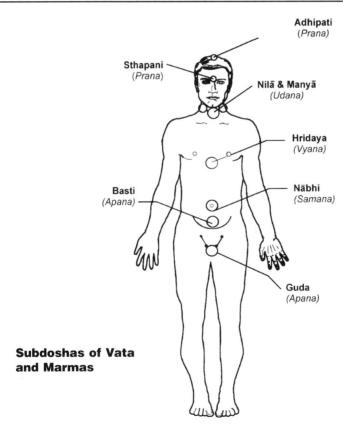

Subdoshas of Vata and Marmas

Pitta Subtypes and Marma Points	
1. Sadhaka Pitta	Simanta, Adhipati and Hridaya marmas (on the head and heart) are related to Sadhaka Pitta and the digestion of knowledge and experience.
2. Alochaka Pitta	Kurcha, Kurchashira, Sthapani and Apanga marmas are related to Alochaka Pitta (seeing power of the eyes) and visual acuity.
3. Bhrajaka Pitta	Nila, Manya, Talahridaya, Amsa and Katikataruna marmas are related to Bhrajaka Pitta and digestion of light and heat at the level of the skin.
4. Pachaka Pitta	Nabhi (navel), Apastambha, Kurchashira and Indrabasti marmas are related to Pachaka Pitta and the digestive system.
5. Ranjaka Pitta	Nabhi (navel), Kurpara (elbow), Janu (knee) and Kukundara marmas are related to Ranjaka Pitta (digestive power at the level of the blood) and the liver.

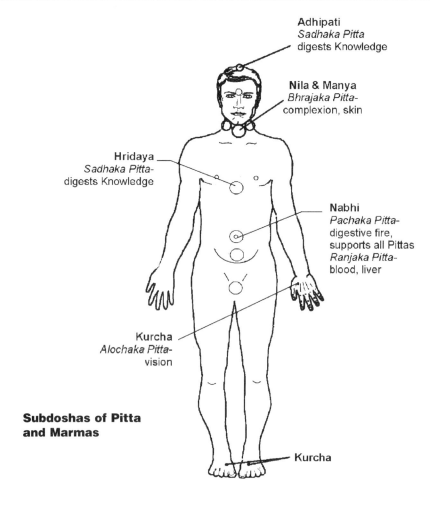

Adhipati
Sadhaka Pitta
digests Knowledge

Nila & Manya
Bhrajaka Pitta-
complexion, skin

Hridaya
Sadhaka Pitta-
digests Knowledge

Nabhi
Pachaka Pitta-
digestive fire,
supports all Pittas
Ranjaka Pitta-
blood, liver

Kurcha
Alochaka Pitta-
vision

**Subdoshas of Pitta
and Marmas**

Kurcha

Kapha Subtypes and Marma Points	
1. Tarpaka Kapha	Adhipati and Simanta on the head and Hridaya (heart) marmas are related with Tarpaka Kapha (emotional contentment). So are Shringataka and Krikatika marmas on the head and neck.
2. Bodhaka Kapha	Shringataka, Manya and Phana marmas on the face and neck are related to Bodhaka Kapha (power of taste).
3. Avalambaka Kapha	Hridaya (heart), Stanamula and Talahridaya marmas are related to Avalambaka Kapha (lubrication of the mucous membranes in the chest).
4. Kledaka Kapha	Nabhi (navel) and Apastambha marmas are related with Kledaka Kapha (Kapha digestive secretions). So is Kurchashira on the hands and feet.
5. Sleshaka Kapha	Janu (knee), Kurpara (elbow), Manibandha (wrist), Gulpha (ankle) and Katikataruna (hip) marmas are related with Sleshaka Kapha (lubrication of the joints).

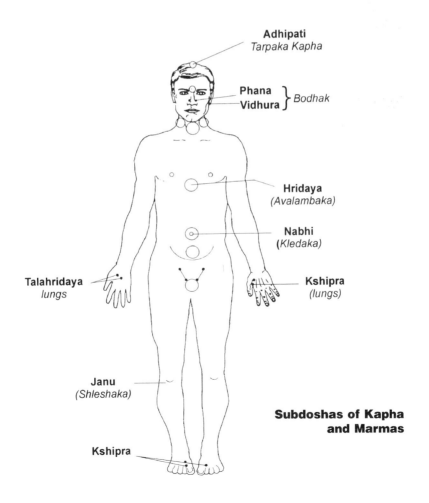

Subdoshas of Kapha and Marmas

3. Channel Systems and Marma Points

The following are a few key marmas relating to the different channel systems. Others are listed in the table of marmas.

1. Pranavaha Srotas— respiratory system, lungs, heart	Talahridaya, Kshipra, Hridaya (heart), Phana, Sthapani
2. Annavaha Srotas— digestive system, g.i. tract	Nabhi (navel), Indrabasti, Kurchashira
3. Udakavaha Srotas—water-metabolism system, pancreas	Apastambha, Kurpara, Janu, Basti, Urvi, Bahvi
4. Rasavaha Srotas—plasma and lymphatic system, heart, skin	Hridaya (heart), Kshipra, Stanamula, Lohitaksha, Amsaphalaka, Nila
5. Raktavaha Srotas—circulatory system, blood, heart, liver	Hridaya (heart), Nabhi (navel), Kurpara (elbow), Brihati, Janu (knee), Lohitaksha, Sira Matrika
6. Mamsavaha Srotas— muscular system	Kurchashira, Kakshadhara, Stanamula, Stanarohita, Guda (anus)
7. Medavaha Srotas— adipose system	Basti (bladder) Katikataruna, Nitamba
8. Asthivaha Srotas— skeletal system	Kukundara, Katikataruna, Janu (knee) Manibandha, Simanta
9. Majjavaha Srotas— nervous system, brain	Adhipati, Simanta, Sthapani, Apalapa, Apastambha, Shringataka
10. Shukravaha Srotas— reproductive system, testes, uterus	Guda (anus), Vitapa (perineum), Gulpha (ankle), Basti (lower abdomen)
11. Mutravaha Srotas— urinary system, kidneys, urinary bladder	Basti (bladder), Guda (anus), Kukundara
12. Purishavaha Srotas— excretory system, colon	Guda (anus), Parshvasandhi, Shankha
13. Swedavaha Srotas— sweating system, skin	Nila, Manya, Katikataruna, Stanarohita
14. Manavaha Srotas— the mind	Adhipati, Simanta, Sthapani, Hridaya (heart)
15. Artavavaha Srotas— menstrual system	Basti (bladder), Guda (anus), Nabhi (navel), Katikataruna, Kukundara
16. Stanyavaha Srotas— lactation system	Hridaya (heart), Stanamula, Stanarohita, Nitamba

Strategies of Marma Therapy/Marma Formulas

Marma therapy is not limited to the treatment of single marmas, however important this can be. Several marmas are usually treated during a session. The number and sequence of marmas treated will determine the nature and effects of the therapy. Naturally, the development of marma formulas, like that of herbal formulas, can be complex. However, using the above correlations one can combine different marmas to treat specific doshas, subdoshas or channel-systems out of balance. Generally three to seven marmas is a good number to consider, focusing on one as the most important or central marma for the formula.

One method is to select marmas from each section of the body like the arms, legs, front of the body, back of the body and head. This can be combined with overall body massage. For example, one can treat Vata in a comprehensive manner through marma therapy on Adhipati (head), Amsa (back of the neck), Guda (anus), Talahridaya (palm of the hand) and Talahridaya (sole of the foot).

Or one can focus on key regions of the subdoshas. For example, one can treat Sadhaka Pitta (Pitta in the nervous system) through marma therapy on Simanta (skull) and Hridaya (heart) marmas. For another example, one can treat Sleshaka Kapha (lubrication of the joints) by doing marma therapy on the main joint marmas: Janu (knee), Kurpara (elbow), Manibandha (wrist), Gulpha (ankle) and Katikataruna (hip).

One can treat the channel-systems in the same manner. For example, to open the Pranavaha Srotas or respiratory/energy system, one can treat Kshipra (hand), Talahridaya (hand), Hridaya (heart), Phana (nostrils) and Adhipati (head) marmas.

Another important principle to consider is that it is generally good to treat the corresponding marmas on both the right and left sides of the body or on both the upper and lower extremities. For example, when treating Kshipra (hand), make sure to treat both right and left points and also Kshipra on the foot. An exception to this is if one is trying to correct an energy imbalance on the right and left sides of the body or on the upper and lower portions of the body. Then one must focus on stimulating marmas on the side or portion of the body requiring energization, while either not treating or sedating the marmas on the opposite side.

These are only a few suggestions. Marma formulas are an advanced topic usually taught in a clinical setting and requiring extensive Ayurvedic knowledge and training by the student.

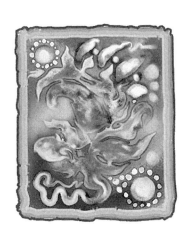

CHAPTER 8

Table of Marmas: Marmas on the Arms and Hands

11 Marma Regions and 22 Points

The hands and arms contain a number of important marma points for the reception and expression of Prana, particularly for Vyana Vayu (the outward-moving pranic force), which they convey through the sense of touch. Such peripheral points on the body impact the circulation of energy in the internal organs and in the spine as well as the arms and leg positions where they are located. They are easy to reach and manipulate for treatment purposes, which makes them very important in marma therapy.

Marmas on the hands are the basis for therapeutic touch. Their energy should be kept strong and clear for those who wish to project their healing power on to others. Treating these specific marmas goes along well with general massage of the arms and hands.

Marmas on the arms have two points, one for each arm. Generally, marmas on the right arm or solar side of the body are better for increasing heat, promoting circulation and improving digestion. They stimulate bodily activities, increasing Agni (fire) and the Pitta functions of the body. Marmas on the left arm or lunar side of the body are better for cooling action, reducing inflammation and building tissue. They have a calming effect, increasing the Kapha or watery functions of the body.

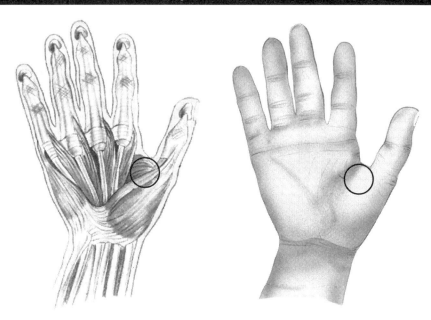

Kshipra hand marma

Kshipra (hand)

Description	
Name	Kshipra (quick; reflecting its immediate effect)
Number	2 marma points, one on each hand
Type	Ligament (Snayu)
Size	1/2 anguli (finger unit)
Site	Situated between the thumb and index finger, located bilaterally on the dorsal and palmar surfaces of the hand in the web formed by the dorsal interosseous muscle between the first and second metacarpal bones. *Note:* (The sites between the other fingers also have important therapeutic properties. They can be regarded as secondary Kshipra points and treated in a similar manner).
Controls	Controls plasma and respiratory systems (Rasavaha and Pranavaha Srotamsi), heart, lungs and Avalambaka Kapha (lubrication of heart and lungs), Prana and Vyana Vayus.
Anatomical Structures	Flexor pollicis brevis, oblique and transverse head of adductor pollicis muscle. Branches of median nerve, dorsal metacarpal

	artery and superficial palmar arch supplying blood to the fingers.
Qualities Relative to Injury	Kalantara Pranahara (Long-term Death-Causing) type marma. Both fiery and watery in degree of vulnerability.
Symptoms If Injured	Loss of adduction and flexion of thumb, and bleeding from the palmar arch.

Treatment

Massage, Acupressure and Aroma Therapy	Apply marma massage to the area, using a strong circular motion for about five minutes. This is also a good marma for acupressure to promote circulation, increase energy flow and get the Prana moving throughout the body as a whole. Use Amrita Taila, plain sesame oil or mustard oil as massage oils. Use spicy aromatic oils like eucalyptus, cinnamon, sage or artemisia to open the energy and relieve pain. Apply powders of calamus or ginger for similar purposes.
Acupuncture (Suchi-karma)	For tingling, numbness, erysipelas, gout, calceneal spur, psoriasis or cracked hands; acupuncture should be done two anguli (finger units) proximal to the site.
Treatment If Injured	Generally apply an ice pack. When there is burning sensation, apply ghee (clarified butter) or, if the sensation is more internal, use sandalwood oil.

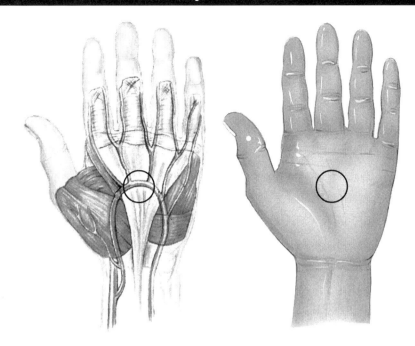

Talahridaya hand marma

Talahridaya (hand)

Description	
Name	Talahridaya (heart or center of the palm)
Number	2 marma points, one on each hand
Type	Muscle (Mamsa)
Size	1/2 anguli (finger unit)
Site	Situated in the center of the palm, facing the root of the middle finger (center of the palmar surface of the hand superficial to the third metacarpo-phalangeal joint).
Controls	An important point for energy circulation for the entire body that is helpful for all around health and balance. Controls respiratory system (Pranavaha Srotas), heart, lungs, Bhrajaka Pitta (circulation and heat reception on the skin) and Avalambaka Kapha (lubrication of heart and lungs). Controls Yashasvati Nadi (right hand) and Hastijihva Nadi (left hand) along with Vyana Vayu (power of circulation), particularly

	in the upper half of the body (above the navel). Also controls the hands as a motor organ.
Anatomical Structures	Tendon of flexor digitorum profundus, lumbricalis and extensor digitorum. Muscle tissue of tunica media of superficial and deep palmar arch. Interossei muscle. Branches of the median nerve.
Qualities Relative to Injury	Kalantara Pranahara (Long-term Death-Causing) marma. Both fiery and watery in degree of vulnerability.
Symptoms If Injured	Loss of flexion and extension of the second, third and fourth fingers and adduction of second, third and fourth metacarpals. Bleeding may lead to pain, shock or infection.

Treatment

Massage, Acupressure and Aroma Therapy	Apply marma massage to the area, using a strong circular motion for about five minutes or until the energy in the hand is released. This is also a good marma for acupressure for opening up the healing energy of the hands. It is often a sore point in most people. Use Narayan Taila, sesame or almond oil for massage. Use spicy aromatic oils like eucalyptus, camphor orelecampane for clearing Pranavaha Srotas (respiratory system). For Vyana Vayu (pranic circulation) and to energize the hands, use penetrating aromatic oils like eucalyptus, cinnamon or camphor. This is great for massage practitioners to prepare themselves for treatment, enhancing the power of therapeutic touch. Rubbing the palms together quickly for a few seconds energizes this point. Once the palms feel warm, they can be placed on other marmas for healing purposes, including over the eyes for calming Pitta or over the ears to calm Vata. Aromatic oils like cinnamon, cardamom, saffron and ginger applied at this point are good for stimulating the heart.
Meditation and Yoga	A good point of concentration and meditation for bringing in positive healing energies and Prana from the external environment and for releasing negative energy and stress.
Treatment If Injured	Although it is a muscle marma, injury to nearby vessels can cause bleeding. To stop bleeding, apply ice to the area. Plain ghee is good for healing the area or the special Ayurvedic formula Shatadhauta Ghrita. Use turmeric and licorice powders made into a paste along with a little castor oil for healing purposes.

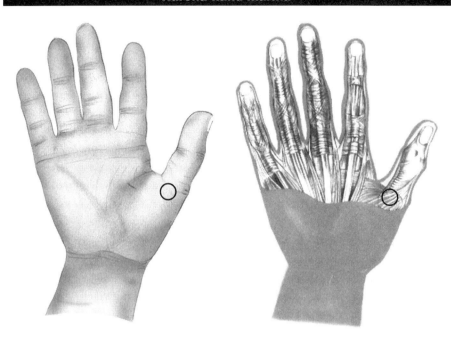

Kurcha hand marma

Kurcha (hand)

Description	
Name	Kurcha (a knot or bundle, of the muscles at the base of the thumb)
Number	2 marma points, one on each hand
Type	Ligament (Snayu)
Size	4 anguli (finger units)
Site	The main point is situated one anguli (finger unit) distal from the wrist joint at the base of the thumb joint (first metacarpo-pha langeal joint), proximal to Kshipra marma, but the entire marma covers a large area. Its large size of four angulis can be explained in that the marma includes the joints of the other fingers as well, which can be regarded as secondary Kurcha points.
Controls	Controls Alochaka Pitta (seeing function of the eyes), overall sensory acuity and Prana Vayu (overall pranic and nerve energy, particularly to the head). An important point for Prana and Vata.

Anatomical Structures	Tendon of extensor digitorum, extensor indicis, tendon of extensor carpi radialis bravis and longus and flexor digitorum sublimus and profundus. Branches of median nerve.
Qualities Relative to Injury	Vaikalyakara (Disability-Causing) type marma. Watery in degree of vulnerability.
Symptoms If Injured	Injury may impair coordination of the carpal and metacarpal joints, extension and abduction of the wrist and cause distortion of the hand.

Treatment	
Massage, Acupressure and Aroma Therapy	Follow usual massage procedures. The central area of this marma is good for acupressure, which also stimulates the mind. For controlling Alochaka Pitta (seeing function of the eyes) massage with sandalwood oil, Brahmi Taila, Shatadhauta Ghrita or plain ghee. Use cooling and sweet aromatic oils like sandalwood, rose, chamomile and lotus. For opening the energy and stimulating Prana use aromatic oils like camphor, mint or cloves. This also helps to keep Vata from getting stagnant.
Treatment If Injured	Apply a supportive bandage to minimize pain. Use turmeric paste or aloe gel for minor injury.

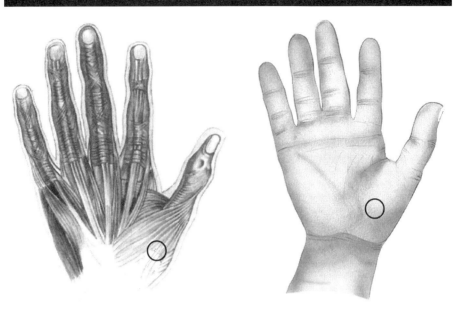

Kurchashira hand marma

Kurchashira (hand)

Description	
Name	Kurchashira (the head of Kurcha)
Number	2 marma points (one on each hand)
Type	Ligament (Snayu)
Size	1 anguli (finger unit)
Site	The root of the thumb just above the wrist. Distal to Manibandha, situated two angulis (finger units) proximal to Kurcha, or between Kurcha and Manibandha, first car-pometacarpal joint distal to the trapezium.
Controls	Controls Alochaka Pitta (seeing power of the eyes), Agni (digestive power), stomach, Pachaka Pitta, Kledaka Kapha and Samana Vayu (forms of Pitta, Kapha and Vata govern-ing digestion). Also influences the head, mind and nervous systems, calming Vata. The thumb is regarded as manifestation of Agni, not simply

	as the power of digestion but also as the power of Prana and as the soul itself. This is an important Agni point for controlling these different forms of fire.
Anatomical Structures	Tendon of flexor carpi radialis, tendon of abductor pollicis longus, tendon of extensor carpi radialis longus, tendon of extensor pollicis longus and brevis.
Qualities Relative to Injury	Rujakara (Pain-causing) type marma. Both airy and fiery in degree of vulnerability.
Symptoms If Injured	Impairment of the flexion and abduction of the wrist, bleeding from the radial artery and pain due to injury to the radial nerve.
Treatment	
Massage, Acupressure and Aroma Therapy	Follow usual massage procedures using a strong massage, particularly with your thumb until the energy in the thumb is released. This is also a good marma for acupressure and helps increase Prana and stimulate Agni in the body overall. For controlling Alochaka Pitta (seeing power of the eyes) use Amalaki Taila, Brahmi Taila, coconut or sunflower oils. Use cooling aromatic oils like sandalwood, rose or khus. For Agni and digestion, use stimulating aromatic oils like ginger, cinnamon, cloves or cardamom. For clearing the mind, use oils like calamus, myrrh or camphor. For calming Vata use oils like sandalwood, valerian or jatamamsi.
Treatment If Injured	Apply turmeric paste or aloe gel for minor injury.

Manibandha marma

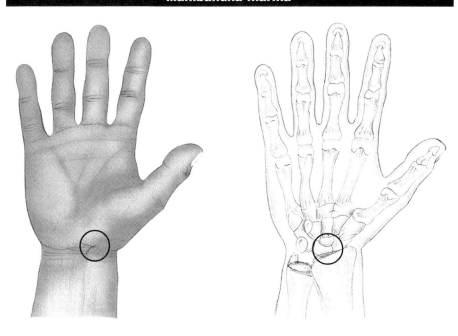

Manibandha

Description	
Name	Manibandha (bracelet)
Number	2 marma points (one on each wrist)
Type	Joint (Sandhi)
Size	2 anguli (finger units)
Site	The wrist, with the main point one-half anguli (finger units) lateral to the center of the wrist joint (anterior radial wrist crease in the well formed by the juncture of the radius with the scaphoid/lunate carpal bones). The site opposite, on the back of the wrist, is also important. Both points can be treated together. The overall marma is medium in size and covers the central part of the wrist joint as a whole.
Controls	Controls skeletal system (Asthivaha Srotas) and movement of hands, Sleshaka Kapha (lubrication of the joints) and Vyana Vayu (peripheral circulation).

Anatomical Structures	Wrist joint. Radio-ulnar and radio-carpal ligaments. Radial and median nerve and artery.
Qualities Relative to Injury	Rujakara (Pain-causing) type marma. Both airy and fiery in degree of vulnerability.
Symptoms If Injured	Loss of flexion, extension, adduction and abduction of the hand. Injury can also cause weakening, discoordination, dislocation and distortion of the hand.

Treatment	
Massage, Acupressure and Aroma Therapy	Follow usual massage procedures with moderate strength until the energy in the wrist is released. The central area of this marma is also a good marma for acupressure for increasing energy flow to the hand. For controlling Asthivaha Srotas (skeletal system) and Sleshaka Kapha, use Sahachara Taila, Ashwagandha Taila, sesame oil or almond oil. Use penetrating and healing aromatic oils like angelica, birch, myrrh, guggul or wintergreen which relieve joint pain and swelling.
Acupuncture (suci karma)	In case of cervical lymphadenitis, perform acupuncture on the point two anguli (finger units) distal to the marma.
Treatment If Injured	For dislocation or fracture apply a bandage to the wrist joint. When there is a simple injury without fracture, bathe the area in warm ghee or sesame oil.

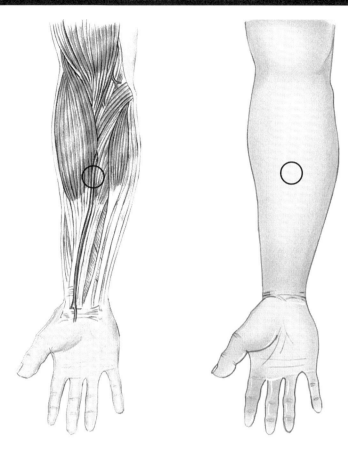

Indrabasti arm marma

Indrabasti (arm)

Description	
Name	Indrabasti (Indra's arrow or a superior type of arrow; owing to the shape of the muscles in the region of the mid-forearm. Basti also means bladder in other contexts.)
Number	2 marma points, one on each forearm
Type	Muscle (Mamsa)
Size	1/2 anguli (finger unit)
Site	Center of the forearm, slightly at the lateral aspect where the radial artery passes (anterior forearm midline between the elbow and wrist crease in the belly of the flexor carpi radialis superficial to the interosseus membrane).

Controls	Controls digestive system (Annavaha Srotas), Agni (digestive fire), Samana Vayu (balancing Prana), Pachaka Pitta (digestive juices) and small intestine. Has an effect on the plasma (Rasa Dhatu) as well.
Anatomical Structures	Flexor pollicis longus, extensor carpi radialis, brachioradialis and pronator teres muscles. Radial and median nerve, radial artery and tributaries of cephalic vein.
Qualities Relative to Injury	Kalantara Pranahara (Long-term Death-Causing) type marma. Both fiery and watery in degree of vulnerability.
Symptoms If Injured	The important structure at this marma is the radial artery. Injury may lead to distortion of the hand resulting in 'Volkmann's contracture'. It may also cause paralysis of the forearm or severe bleeding.
Treatment	
Massage, Acupressure and Aroma Therapy	Apply marma massage to the area, using a strong circular motion for about five minutes. This is also a good marma for acupressure. For stimulation of Agni (digestive fire), use Mahamasha Taila, mustard or sesame oils. For controlling the small intestine and Annavaha Srotas (digestive system), use warm spicy aromatic oils like anise, fennel, ginger or cardamom. Calamus oil is good here for promoting circulation in both the digestive system and through the plasma.
Treatment If Injured	The same as Kshipra.

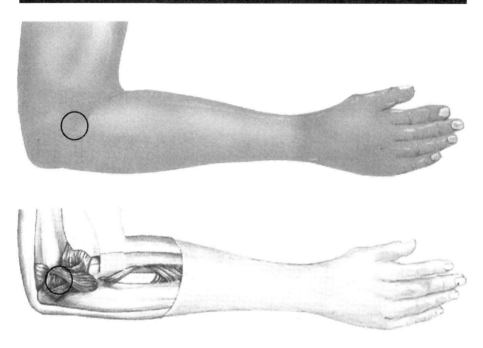

Kurpara marma

Kurpara

Description	
Name	Kurpara (elbow-joint)
Number	2 marma points, one on each arm
Type	Joint (Sandhi)
Size	3 anguli (finger units)
Site	The elbow joint as a whole, a large marma. The main point is at the outside (trochlear notch, lateral elbow superficial to radial collateral ligament). However, the corresponding point on the inside and the point immediately behind the elbow joint are also important points.
Controls	Controls blood and circulatory system (Raktavaha Srotas), Samana Vayu (balancing Prana), Ranjaka Pitta (coloring of the blood and bile) and Udakavaha Srotas (water-metabolism). Marma on right elbow controls the liver and Ranjaka Pitta. Marma on left elbow controls the spleen, pancreas and Udakavaha Srotas.

Anatomical Structures	Elbow join, ligament capsule, ulnar, radial and annular radial collateral ligaments, median nerve and branches. Brachial artery, tributaries of cephalic and median cubital vein. Supinator, extensor carpi radialis, biceps, triceps and pronator teres muscles.
Qualities Relative to Injury	Vaikalyakara (Disability-Causing) type marma. Watery in degree of vulnerability.
Symptoms If Injured	Injury will cause bleeding and damage the function of the forearm.

Treatment

Massage, Acupressure and Aroma Therapy	For liver diseases, massage the right Kurpara marma. Use Padmakadi Taila, Manjishtadi Taila, Brahmi Taila, ghee or safflower oils for massage. Use blood-cleansing aromatic oils like coriander, myrrh, wormwood, saffron or turmeric. For diseases of spleen and pancreas, massage the left Kurpara marma with Manjishtadi Taila, safflower oil or sesame oil. Use spicy aromatic oils like ginger, cardamom, myrrh or turmeric. For acupressure, the points on the outside and the inside, in front and behind the elbow, are also good and can be worked on with some strength.
Heat Application (Agni-karma)	For enlargement of the liver, select a sensitive point on the right marma and apply heat with a metal probe. For enlargement of the spleen, use a sensitive point on the left marma. The heat applied should be mild. The procedure can be repeated every alternate day for seven days.
Blood-letting (Sira Vedha)	For liver disorders, blood-letting should be done from the right cubital vein. For spleen disorders, it should be done from the left cubital vein. Only small amounts of blood should be taken and the wound covered with turmeric powder and aloe gel or other suitable disinfectant.
Acupuncture (Suchi-karma)	For brachial neuralgia, cervical spondylitis, tingling or numbness of the palm, acupuncture should be done on the point four anguli (finger units) either proximal or distal to Kurpara marma.
Treatment If Injured	Apply a cross type bandage to the area. Use herbs like turmeric and myrrh internally to promote healing, or guggul and ashwagandha as tonics if there is injury to the bone.

Ani arm marma

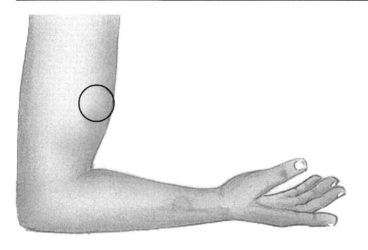

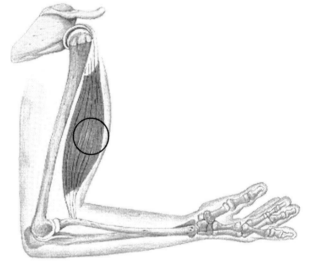

Ani (arm)

Description	
Name	Ani (the point of a needle)
Number	2 marma points, one on each arm
Type	Ligament and Tendon (Snayu)
Size	1/2 anguli (finger unit)

Site	In the medial aspect of the arm, two anguli (finger units) proximal to the medial epicondyle of the humerus.
Controls	Controls Udakavaha Srotas (water-metabolism system), pancreas and kidneys.
Anatomical Structures	Biceps and coracobrachial muscles. Ulnar and median nerves. Lower end of the humerus. Brachial artery and vein.
Qualities Relative to Injury	Vaikalyakara (Disability-Causing) type marma. Watery in degree of vulnerability.
Symptoms If Injured	Injury to this marma impairs extension of the arm, as well as the drawing of the arm forward and inward. Injury to the nerve may cause complete paralysis of the arm. Injury to the artery may cause severe bleeding.
Treatment	
Massage, Acupressure and Aroma Therapy	An easy area to reach for massage. Follow usual massage or acupressure procedures. For controlling Udakavaha Srotas (water-metabolism system) massage with Amalaki Taila or plain mustard oil. Use Kapha-removing aromatic oils like ginger, cardamom, parsley or juniper.
Treatment If Injured	A paste of aloe gel and turmeric can be used for minor injury.

Bahvi (Urvi, arm) marma

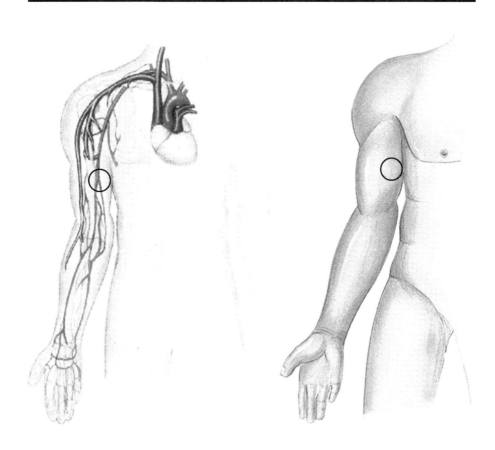

Bahvi (Urvi, arm)

Description	
Name	Bahvi (what relates to the arm) or Urvi (the wide region of the upper arm)
Number	2 marma points, one on each arm
Type	Vessel (Sira)
Size	1 anguli (finger unit)
Site	In the radial aspect of the upper arm about four and a half anguli (finger units) from the medial epicondyle.

Controls	Controls plasma and water-metabolism (Rasavaha and Udakavaha Srotamsi), Vyana Vayu and governs healthy tissue growth.
Anatomical Structures	Brachial artery and vein. Lymph vessel drainage to axillary group of glands. Median and ulnar nerves. Biceps and triceps muscles.
Qualities Relative to Injury	Vaikalyakara (Disability-Causing) type of marma. Watery in degree of vulnerability.
Symptoms If Injured	Damage to the artery causes bleeding. Injury may cause impairment of the function of flexion and extension of the arm.

Treatment

Massage, Acupressure and Aroma Therapy	Apply marma massage to the area, using a strong circular motion for about five minutes. Acupressure also works well here for improving lymphatic circulation. Massage with plain sesame, almond or mustard oils to warm the region. For controlling Rasavaha Srotas (lymphatic system) use drying aromatic oils like camphor, cardamom, bayberry or mint. For improving circulation use stimulating aromatic oils like cinnamon, thyme or ginger.
Treatment If Injured	For bleeding apply ice to the site and if necessary a pressure bandage. Use hemostatic herbs like yarrow, mullein, nagakeshara or plantain.

Lohitaksha arm marma

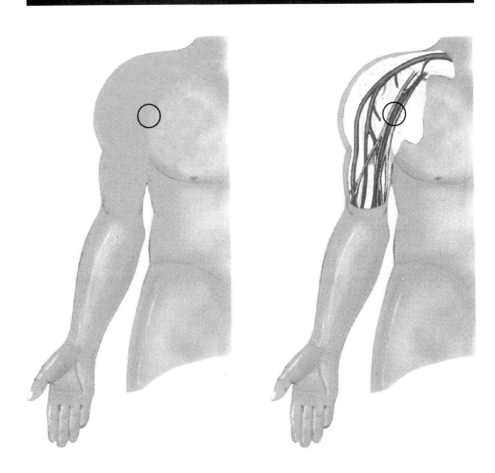

Lohitaksha (arm)

Description	
Name	Lohitaksha (red-jointed; the lower frontal insert of the shoulder joint)
Number	2 marma points (one on each shoulder)
Type	Vessel (Sira)
Size	1/2 anguli (finger unit)
Site	Center of the armpit or axillary fossa through which axillary artery passes, anterior aspect of axillary crease.

Controls	Controls plasma and lymphatic system (Rasavaha Srotas), blood (Raktavaha Srotas) and Vyana Vayu (peripheral circulation), particularly to the legs.
Anatomical Structures	Axillary artery and vein. Lymph vessel drainage to axillary group of glands. Median and ulnar nerves. Latissimus dorsi, pectoralis major and minor, coracobrachial and subscapular muscles.
Qualities Relative to Injury	Vaikalyakara (Disability-Causing) marma. Watery in degree of vulnerability.
Symptoms If Injured	Damage to the axillary vessels can cause hemorrhage. Injury to the muscles may cause loss of function of the humerus.

Treatment

Massage, Acupressure, and Aroma Therapy	Follow usual marma massage procedures. This is a good marma for acupressure, which will help drain the lymphatics and release muscular tension. For controlling Rasavaha Srotas (lymphatic system), use Bilvadi Taila, mustard oil or sesame oil for massage. Use Kapha-reducing aromatic oils like eucalyptus, cinnamon, mint or cardamom. For controlling Raktavaha Srotas (blood), use Amla Taila or sesame oil and aromatic oils like saffron, rose, myrrh or cinnamon.
Treatment If Injured	If there is bleeding apply ice and if necessary pressure bandage. Use hemostatic herbs internally like yarrow, mullein or nagakeshara. As food therapy give a mixture of banana, milk and sugar to restore body fluids if necessary.

Kakshadhara marma

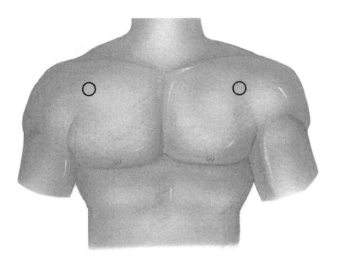

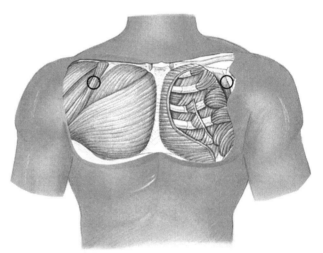

Kakshadhara

Description	
Name	Kakshadhara (what upholds the flanks; near the top of the shoulder joint)
Number	2 marma points (one on each shoulder)
Type	Ligament (Snayu)
Size	1 anguli (finger unit)

Site	Two anguli (finger units) below the point joining the lateral one-third and medial two-thirds of clavicle, where the median nerve is situated, or lateral edge of the tip of the coracoid process of the shoulder girdle.
Controls	Controls muscular system (Mamsavaha Srotas), shoulders, bodily posture and Vyana Vayu.
Anatomical Structures	Pectoralis major and minor as well as intercostal muscles. Median nerve. Lymph vessel drainage to axillary glands. Axillary artery and vein.
Qualities Relative to Injury	Vaikalyakara (Disability-Causing) type of marma Watery in degree of vulnerability.
Symptoms If Injured	Injury may cause impairment of movement, downward and forward drawing of the arm, and depression of the shoulder joint. Nerve injury may lead to paralysis of the hand, wasting of the muscles or infection.
Treatment	
Massage, Acupressure and Aroma Therapy	A good marma for relieving muscular tension either through massage or through acupressure. Good for stiff shoulders owing to high Vata. For controlling Mamsavaha Srotas (muscular system) use Mahamasha Taila, Chandan-bala-lakshadi Taila or plain sesame oil. Use aromatic oils like eucalyptus, cinnamon, turmeric, myrrh or saffron which improve circulation to the muscles. A special Ayurvedic oil called Kuzambu Taila (4 parts sesame oil, 2 parts ghee and 1 part castor oil) is very effective here.
Treatment if Injured	Apply castor oil for pain relief.

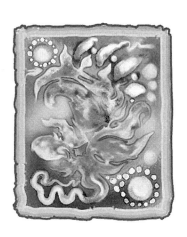

CHAPTER 9

Marmas on the Legs and Feet

11 Regions and 22 Points

The marmas on the legs and feet mirror those on the arms and hands in both number and location, which is why most have the same names. The legs contain important marmas for the reception of Prana from the Earth, which occurs mainly through the feet, and for the projection of Prana through walking and running. This connects the leg marmas both with Vyana Vayu, the outward-moving air that governs movement, and also with Apana Vayu, the downward-moving air that connects us to the force of gravity and governs the processes of elimination and reproduction. Treating these marmas goes along with massage of the legs and the feet.

Marma regions on the legs like those on the arms have two points, one on each leg. Generally, marmas on the right leg or solar side of the body are better for increasing heat, promoting circulation and improving digestion. They stimulate bodily activities, increasing Agni (fire) and the Pitta functions of the body. Marmas on the left leg or lunar side of the body are better for cooling action, reducing inflammation and building tissue. They have a calming effect, increasing the Kapha or watery functions of the body.

Kshipra foot marma

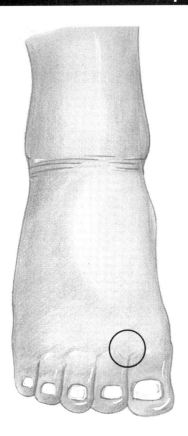 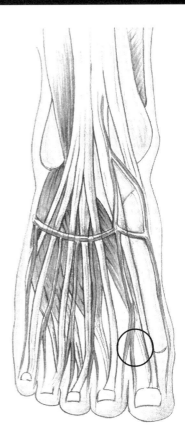

Kshipra (foot)

Description	
Name	Kshipra (quick; reflecting its immediate effect)
Number	2 marma points, one on each foot
Type	Ligament (Snayu)
Size	1/2 anguli (finger unit) in size
Site	In between the big toe and the first toe (web between the first distal phalangeal joint and the second medial phalangeal joints of the foot). *Note:* (The sites between the other toes also have important therapeutic properties.)

Controls	Controls lymphatic and respiratory systems (Rasavaha and Pranavaha Srotamsi), Avalambaka Kapha (lubrication for heart and lungs) and heart and lungs overall.
Anatomical Structures	Adductor hallucis bravis and lumbrical muscles. Posterior tibial nerve. Dorsal metatarsal artery, plantar arch and medial plantar artery. Metatarso-phalangeal joint.
Qualities Relative to Injury	Kalantara Pranahara (Long-term Death-Causing) type marma. Both fiery and watery in degree of vulnerability.
Symptoms If Injured	Injury may impair the functions of adduction and flexion of the great toe. Damage to the artery may cause bleeding, hematoma inside the plantar aponeurosis and toxemia.
Treatment	
Massage, Acupressure and Aroma Therapy	Apply marma massage to the area, using a strong circular motion for about five minutes. This is also a good marma for acupressure for promoting the flow of Prana, particularly in the lower limbs. Use Mahanarayan Taila, sesame oil or almond oil for massage purposes. For opening and clearing the lungs, heart and lymphatics use penetrating aromatic oils like camphor, cinnamon, cardamom, or eucalyptus.
Treatment If Injured	The same as the treatment for Kshipra on the hand.

Talahridaya foot marma

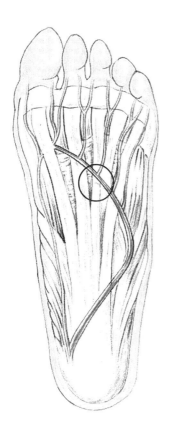
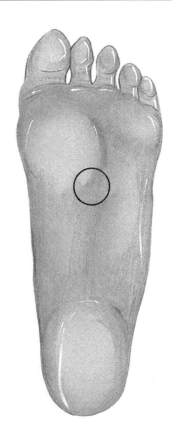

Talahridaya (foot)

Description	
Name	Talahridaya (heart or center of the foot)
Number	2 marma points, one on each foot
Type	Muscle (Mamsa)
Size	1/2 anguli (finger units) in size
Site	Upper center of the sole in line with the root of the third toe. Plantar aspect of the third tarso-metatarsal joint, where the external plantar artery sweeps across the plantar arch of the foot.

Controls	Controls respiratory system (Pranavaha Srotas), Bhrajaka Pitta (circulation and heat reception on the skin), and the feet as a motor organ. Controls Yashasvati Nadi (right foot) and Hastijihva Nadi (left foot) along with Vyana Vayu (power of circulation), particularly for the lower part of the body (below the navel) and Apana Vayu. Controls the earth element in the body as a whole and the feet as a motor organ.
Anatomical Structures	Flexor digitorum brevis and longus muscles. Adductor hallucis, flexor digitorum accessor muscles. Muscle tissue of tunica media of plantar arch. Plantar arch artery and tributaries of cephanous vein.
Qualities Relative to Injury	Kalantara Pranahara (Long-term Death-Causing) type marma. Both fiery and watery in degree of vulnerability.
Symptoms If Injured	Injury may cause impairment of the function of flexion and extension of phalanges and adduction of the great toe. Severe bleeding may occur due to injury to the plantar arch.
Treatment	
Massage, Acupressure and Aroma Therapy	Apply marma massage to the area, using a strong circular motion for about five minutes or until the energy in the foot is released. This is also a good marma for acupressure, which will reduce Vata and control Apana, strengthening the immune system. Use Bala Taila, sesame oil or almond oil to strengthen the feet and calm the nerves. Use diuretic aromatic oils like cedar, Himalayan cedar, parsley or juniper for promoting circulation in the lower body. The application of garlic oil here is very grounding, calming and Vata-reducing. It also strengthens the immune system, the reproductive system and Ojas. Aromatic oils like cinnamon, cardamom, saffron and ginger applied at this point are good for stimulating the heart.
Meditation and Yoga	A good point for meditation to create grounding, calm Vata and to draw in healing energies from the Earth into the body and the circulatory system. It can also be used to release negative energy and stress down into the Earth.
Treatment If Injured	The same as Talahridaya of the hand.

Kurcha foot marma

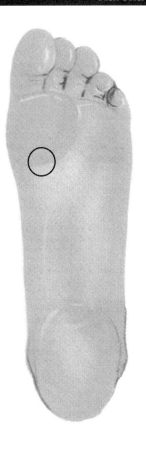 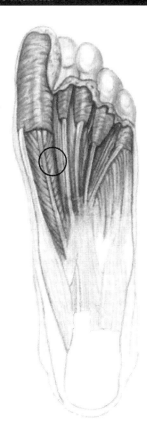

Kurcha (foot)

Description	
Name	Kurcha (a knot or bundle of muscles and tendons)
Number	2 marma points, one on each foot
Type	Ligament (Snayu)
Size	4 anguli (finger units)
Site	The main point is two anguli (finger units) proximal and one-half anguli (finger units) medial to the center of the sole of the foot (web between the first and second metatarsal phalangeal joint), but the entire marma covers a large area. Its large size of four anguli can only be explained if it includes the points at the root of the other toes.

Controls	Controls Alochaka Pitta (seeing power of the eyes), overall sensory acuity and Prana Vayu.
Anatomical Structures	Tendon of flexor hallucis longus and abductor hallucis muscle. Medial plantar nerve. Medial plantar and dorsal metatarsal and arcuate arteries.
Qualities Relative to Injury	Vaikalyakara (Disability-Causing) type marma. Watery in degree of vulnerability.
Symptoms If Injured	Injury may cause damage to the bones and ligaments resulting in discoordination of the muscles of the foot. The shape of the foot may get distorted.
Treatment	
Massage, Acupressure and Aroma Therapy	Follow usual massage procedures. Strong pressure can be used. The center of this marma is good for acupressure for relieving stress and improving mental acuity. For controlling Alochaka Pitta (seeing power of the eyes), use massage oils like Triphala Ghee, Brahmi Taila or plain ghee. Use sweet aromatic oils like sandalwood, rose or chamomile.
Treatment If Injured	The same as Kurcha on the hand.

Kurchashira foot marma

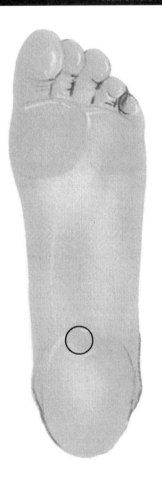
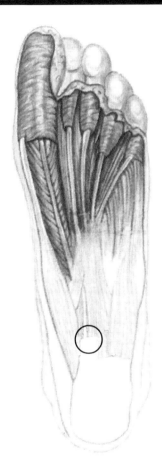

Kurchashira (foot)

Description	
Name	Kurchashira (the head of kurcha)
Number	2 marma points, one on each leg
Type	Ligament (Snayu)
Size	1 anguli (finger units)
Site	Plantar surface of the foot, midpoint on the inferior lateral surface of the calcaneum (os calcis, heel bone).

Controls	Controls muscular system (Mamsavaha Srotas), particularly muscles of the foot, and bodily posture. Like the Kurchashira hand marma is also good for Agni and for digestion.
Anatomical Structures	Peroneous bravis and longus muscles. Peroneal artery and tributaries of short saphanous vein. Peroneal nerve.
Qualities Relative to Injury	Rujakara (Pain-causing) type marma. Both airy and fiery in degree of vulnerability.
Symptoms If Injured	Damage to the ligaments and bone may cause severe pain along with the impairment of the functions of the foot.

Treatment	
Massage, Acupressure and Aroma Therapy	Follow usual massage procedures, using a strong pressure. The center of this marma is good for acupressure for relieving muscular tension and improving the posture. Massage with strengthening and pain-relieving oils like sesame or castor. Special Ayurvedic oils are Durvadi Taila and Ushiradi Taila. Aromatic oils that work on the muscles like saffron, myrrh, guggul or cinnamon are best. For improving Agni and digestion, use stimulating oils like ginger, camphor or garlic.
Heat Application (Agni-karma)	For calcenial spur, it should be done on the nearest sensitive point.
Treatment If Injured	To relieve pain, massage with castor oil or Dashamula Taila. If there is pus formation, use a poultice of comfrey leaves or plantain or a paste of turmeric. A good Ayurvedic preparation is guduchi extract.

Gulpha marma

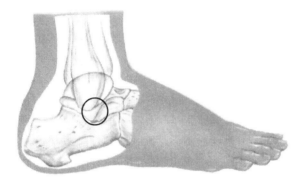

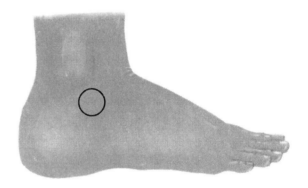

Gulpha

Description	
Name	Gulpha (ankle joint)
Number	2 marma points (one on each ankle)
Type	Joint (Sandhi)
Size	2 anguli (finger units)
Site	The ankle joint, particularly the sensitive point on the inside and below the protuberance of the bone. The point on the outside and below the protuberance of the ankle joint is also good.

Controls	Controls fat, bone and reproductive systems (Medovaha, Asthivaha and Shukravaha Srotamsi), Vyana Vayu (circulation of Prana), Sleshaka Kapha (lubrication of the joints) and movement of the feet
Anatomical Structures	Flexor hallucis longus and bravis, tibilias posterior and flexor digiti longus muscles. Posterior tibial nerve. Posterior tibial artery and vein.
Qualities Relative to Injury	Rujakara (Pain-causing) type marma. Both airy and fiery in degree of vulnerability.
Symptoms If Injured	Injury to the joint will cause swelling and impair the functions of flexion and extension.

Treatment

Massage, Acupressure and Aroma Therapy	Apply marma massage to the area, using a gentle circular motion for about five minutes. For acupressure, use the sensitive point just below the joint on the inside. The point below the joint on the outside can be used as well. For controlling Asthivaha Srotas (skeletal system), use Ashwagandha Taila, Triphaladi Taila, plain sesame oil or almond oil. Use analgesic aromatic oils like myrrh, guggul, angelica and wintergreen. For the reproductive system use aromatic oils like saffron, jasmine or rose for females and nutmeg or musk for males. This will also increase Ojas. For reducing fat, massage with mustard oil and use light aromatic oils like camphor, mint or ginger.
Acupuncture (Suchi-karma)	For tubercular knee, severe pain in the groin, or paralysis of the leg, it should be done on the point four anguli (finger units) above the marma.
Treatment If Injured	The same as Manibandha of the hand.

Indrabasti leg marma

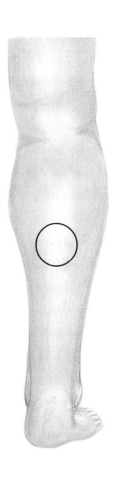 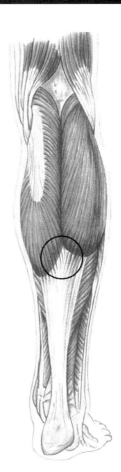

Indrabasti (leg)

Description	
Name	Indrabasti (Indra's arrow or a superior type of arrow; owing to the shape of the muscles in the region of the mid-lower leg. Basti also means bladder in other contexts.)
Number	2 marma points, one on each leg
Type	Muscle (Mamsa)
Size	1/2 anguli (finger unit)

Site	The point at the middle of the line, joining the posterior surface of the calceneum with the center of the popliteal fossa (recess formed between the insertion points of the two gastrocnemius branches into the plantaris tendon).
Controls	Controls digestive system (Annavaha Srotas), Agni (digestive fire), Pachaka Pitta, Samana Vayu, and small intestine.
Anatomical Structures	Gastrocnemius, soleus and plantaris muscles. Peroneal (branch of posterior tibial) and posterior tibial artery and vein. Drainage of lymph vessels to the popletial lymph glands. Posterior tibial nerve.
Qualities Relative to Injury	Kalantara Pranahara (Long-term Death-Causing) type of marma. Both fiery and watery in degree of vulnerability.
Symptoms If Injured	At this vital point, the posterior tibial artery is more important than any other muscle or ligament. Injury may impair the functions of the foot. If the artery is damaged, there will be severe bleeding, shock and collapse.
Treatment	
Massage, Acupressure and Aroma Therapy	Apply marma massage to the area, using a strong circular motion for about five minutes. Acupressure here is also good, particularly for increasing Agni and promoting digestion. For improving the function of small intestine and Annavaha Srotas (digestive system), massage with aromatic oils that stimulate digestion like fennel, ginger, anise or ajwan. For stimulation of Agni, special Ayurvedic formulas are Kshara Taila or Hingutrigunadi Taila containing garlic, asafoetida and rock salt. Or apply warm aromatic oils like ginger, cinnamon or black pepper.
Treatment If Injured	The same as Indrabasti of the hand.

Janu marma

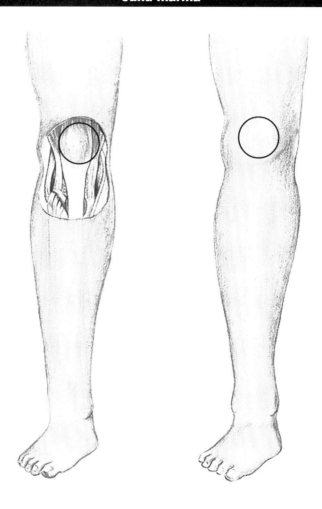

Janu

Description	
Name	Janu (knee joint)
Number	2 marma points (one on each knee)
Type	Joint (Sandhi)
Size	3 anguli (finger units)
Site	The knee joint as a whole, a large marma. Various sensitive points around the knee can be used. The front point is usually

	used, but the back point can be used as well, as can the points on the outside and inside.
Controls	Controls Sleshaka Kapha (lubrication of the joints) and circulation to the legs. The right knee marma controls the liver and Ranjaka Pitta (coloring of blood and bile); the left knee marma controls the spleen and pancreas and Udakavaha Srotas (water-metabolism).
Anatomical Structures	Knee joint. Posterior cruciate ligament, oblique posterior ligament. Plantaris and gastrocenemius muscles. Popliteal artery and vein. Femur, tibia and patella bones. Medial popliteal nerve.
Qualities Relative to Injury	Vaikalyakara (Disability-Causing) type marma. Watery in degree of vulnerability.
Symptoms If Injured	Can cause severe pain, edema, difficulty walking and impairment of the functions of the joint.

Treatment	
Massage, Acupressure and Aroma Therapy	Apply marma massage to the area, using a gentle circular motion for about five minutes. The central point of this joint is best for acupressure, but the points immediately above and below the joint can also be good. For improving liver function, massage the marma on the right knee with Nalapamaradi Taila, Brahmi Taila or plain ghee. Use Pitta-reducing aromatic oils like lime, myrrh, wormwood or coriander. For improving spleen function, massage the marma on the left knee with Bhringamalakadi Taila or plain sesame oil. Use Kapha-removing aromatic oils like ginger, lemon or cardamom. Saffron or turmeric oils can be used for either liver or spleen. For treating arthritis of the knees and Sleshaka Kapha use warming massage oils like Ashwagandha Taila or sesame oil and stimulating aromatic oils like eucalyptus, camphor or cinnamon.
Heat Application (Agni-karma)	In sciatica, select a sensitive point four anguli (finger units) proximal or distal to the marma and apply heated metal rod at the point.
Treatment If Injured	Generally the same as per Kurpara (elbow) marma. Camphor or wintergreen oils are good for knee pain.

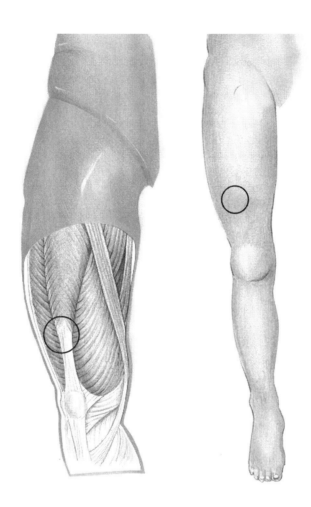

Ani (leg)

Description	
Name	Ani (the point of a needle)
Number	2 marma points, one on each leg
Type	Ligament and Tendon (Snayu)
Size	1/2 anguli (finger unit)

Site	Two anguli (finger units) above the top of the knee joint, and in the middle of the line between the top of the anterior face of the joint and the popliteal surface.
Controls	Controls Udakavaha Srotas (water-metabolism system) and circulation of bodily fluids downward.
Anatomical Structures	Medial and lateral ligaments of the knee joint. Quadriceps muscle and tendon. Femoral artery, tributaries of femoral vein and saphanous nerve.
Qualities Relative to Injury	Vaikalyakara (Disability-Causing) type marma. Watery in degree of vulnerability.
Symptoms If Injured	Injury will cause severe pain and loss of functions of the knee.
Treatment	
Massage, Acupressure and Aroma Therapy	Apply marma massage to the area, using a strong circular motion for about five minutes. Acupressure here will promote the circulation of water and fluids in the body. For controlling Udakavaha Srotas (water-metabolism system) massage with Panchamla Taila, Amalaki Taila or plain sesame or mustard oils. Use water-removing aromatic oils like cardamom, parsley, cedar or ginger.
Treatment If Injured	The same as Ani marma on the hand.

Urvi leg marma

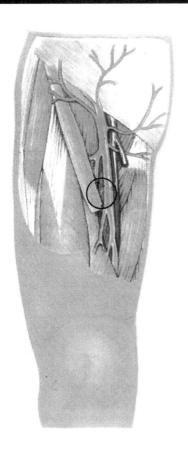 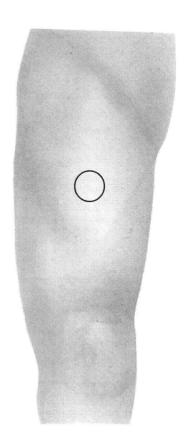

Urvi (leg)

Description	
Name	Urvi (wide; the wide midregion of the thigh)
Number	2 marma points (one on each thigh)
Type	Vessel (Sira)
Size	1 anguli (finger unit)
Site	In the middle of the line joining the center of the inguinal ligament and the medial condyle of the femur where the femoral artery and long saphenous vein pass.

Controls	Controls plasma and water-metabolism (Rasavaha and Udakavaha Srotamsi), Kapha dosha and the water element in the body as a whole.
Anatomical Structures	Femoral artery and vein. Drainage to the superficial inguinal glands. Saphenous nerve. Adductor magnus and rectus femorus muscles.
Qualities Relative to Injury	Vaikalyakara (Disability-Causing) type marma. Watery in degree of vulnerability.
Symptoms If Injured	Injury to the important structures passing through this vital point-artery, nerve and vein-can cause wasting, dysfunction of the muscles and bleeding.

Treatment

Massage, Acupressure and Aroma Therapy	Apply marma massage to the area, using a strong circular motion for about five minutes. Acupressure here aids in weight-reduction and removing Kapha. Strong pressure can be used. For improving the function of Rasavaha Srotas (lymphatic system) massage with Jirakadi Taila (cumin medicated oil) or with plain almond oil or mustard oil. Use diuretic aromatic oils like cedar, juniper, parsley or cardamom to keep the water element in the body flowing properly.
Treatment If Injured	If there is bleeding, apply ice to the area and administer hemostatic herbs that promote the coagulation of blood like turmeric or myrrh. Or apply a pressure bandage to the area.

Lohitaksha leg marma

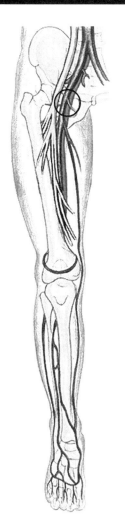 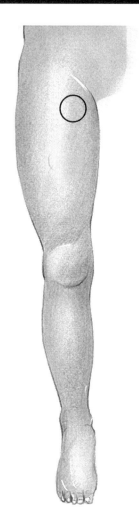

Lohitaksha (leg)

Description	
Name	Lohitaksha (red-jointed; the lower frontal region of the hip joint)
Number	2 marma points, one on each leg
Type	Vessel (Sira)
Size	1/2 anguli (finger unit)

Site	Two anguli (finger units) lateral to the symphysis pubis where the femoral artery passes, in femoral triangle.
Controls	Controls plasma and lymphatic system (Rasavaha Srotas), blood (Raktavaha Srotas), Vyana and Apana Vayus (peripheral and downward movements of energy particularly to the legs).
Anatomical Structures	Femoral artery and tributaries of femoral vein. Femoral nerve. Drainage to the superficial inguinal glands. Psoas major and pectineal muscles.
Qualities Relative to Injury	Vaikalyakara (Disability-Causing) type marma. Watery in degree of vulnerability.
Symptoms If Injured	Injury can cause paralysis of the lower limb and edema of the leg along with deformity and severe pain.
Treatment	
Massage, Acupressure and Aroma Therapy	Follow usual marma massage procedures. Acupressure here aids in draining the nearby lymphatic system. For controlling Rasavaha Srotas (plasma and lymphatics) and it's diseases, massage with Karpuradi (camphor) Taila or with plain mustard oil. Use diaphoretic (sweat-promoting) aromatic oils like basil, sage, cinnamon and eucalyptus. For controlling Raktavaha Srotas (blood) and promoting circulation, use Amla Taila or sesame oil and aromatic oils like saffron, rose, myrrh or cinnamon.
Acupuncture (Suchi-karma)	For treating galaganda (thyroid hypertrophy) select a point one anguli (finger unit) medial to the marma.
Treatment If Injured	The same as Lohitaksha on the hand.

Vitapa marma

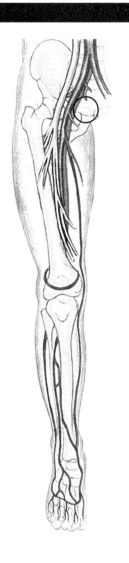 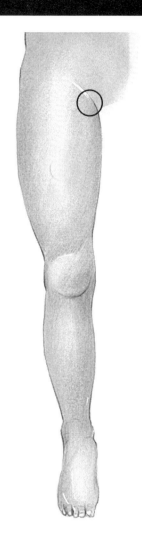

Vitapa

Description	
Name	Vitapa (causing heat or pain; perineum)
Number	2 marma points
Type	Ligament (Snayu)
Size	1 anguli (finger unit)

Site	One anguli (finger unit) lateral to pubic symphysis in the superficial ring through which the spermatic cord passes in men. Inferior aspect of the pubic symphysis.
Controls	Controls reproductive system (Shukravaha Srotas), menstrual system (Artavavaha Srotas), Apana Vayu and Ojas.
Anatomical Structures	In men-external and internal oblique muscles of the abdomen, rectus abdominis muscle, femoral nerve and spermatic cord. In women-round ligament, labia majora and labia minora.
Qualities Relative to Injury	Vaikalyakara (Disability-Causing) type marma. Watery in degree of vulnerability.
Symptoms If Injured	Impotence and sperm deficiency in men. Infertility and menstrual problems for women.

Treatment

Massage, Acupressure and Aroma Therapy	Acupressure is often easier at this narrow region than is massage which must be done carefully. But take care as the region can be sensitive. For controlling Shukravaha Srotas (reproductive system) massage with Masha Taila, Kumkumadi (saffron) Taila, almond oil or sesame oil. Use aromatic oils that strengthen the reproductive system and increase Ojas like jasmine, gardenia or saffron for women and musk (floral hibiscus), nutmeg or cloves for men.
Acupuncture (Suchi-karma)	For treating infections in genital tract and oligospermia, select a point two anguli (finger units) medial to the marma. For treating hydrocele, select a point posterior to the scrotum.
Yoga and Meditation	A good point for concentration and meditation to aid in the control of sexual energy. The yogic practice of Mulabandha, which involves tightening the muscles of the perineum is good for this marma.
Treatment If Injured	The same as Kakshadhara marma on the hand.

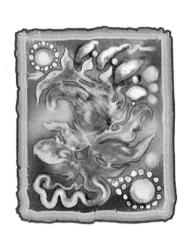

CHAPTER 10

Marmas on the Abdomen and Chest

8 Regions and 12 Points

Marmas on the front side of the body, the abdomen and chest, are fewer in number but very important as this area houses our main internal organs. Some are large marma regions like the heart and the navel. Though generally regarded as only one marma region, they can have many smaller marma points, trigger points or sensitive zones around them that can be used for therapeutic purposes.

These marmas on the front of the body are good for working on the internal organs connected to them. They are also good for working on their corresponding chakras, affecting them through their locations on the front of the body. The front of the body includes the main sites of the accumulation of the doshas in the large intestine (Vata), small intestine (Pitta) and stomach (Kapha) and can be used to promote the elimination of the doshas from these locations. Treating these regions is essential for proper digestion and for detoxification.

Guda marma

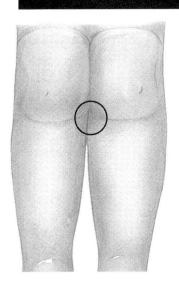
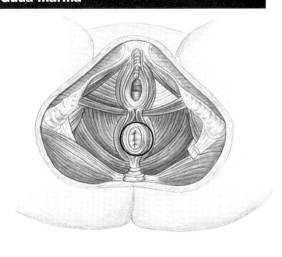

Guda

Description	
Name	Guda (anus)
Number	1 marma point
Type	Muscle (Mamsa)
Size	4 anguli (finger units)
Site	Anus and surrounding area, a large marma.
Controls	Controls the first chakra (Muladhara), Alambusha nadi, Apana Vayu, the channels of excretory, urinary, reproductive and menstrual systems (Purishavaha, Mutravaha, Shukravaha and Artavavaha Srotamsi) as well as the testes and ovaries. Relates to Vata's site of accumulation in the large intestine.
Anatomical Structures	Sphincter ani internus and externus, corrugator cutis ani muscles. Rectal plexus of nerves. Inferior rectal artery and vein.
Qualities Relative to Injury	Sadya Pranahara (Immediate Death-Causing) type marma. Fiery in degree of vulnerability.
Symptoms If Injured	Injury to the sphincter muscles results in loss of control of the anus. Similarly sudden dilation can cause a reflex stoppage of heart.

Treatment	
Massage, Acupressure and Aroma Therapy	Be careful not to get any aromatic oils on the mucus membranes as this will cause pain and a burning sensation. Apply these to the surrounding area only. The point at the base of the spine (corresponding to the first chakra) is probably the best region of this marma for massage, acupressure and aroma therapy. To reduce Vata, use a gentle massage of warm sesame or medicated sesame oils (tailas like Dashamula Taila). For improving functions of Mutravaha Srotas (urinary system) massage with mustard oil. Also use diuretic aromatic oils like juniper, birch or parsley. For aiding menstruation use aromatic oils like saffron, myrrh or pennyroyal, which strengthen and stimulate the female reproductive system. For controlling obesity, use Asana-bilvadi Taila or use weight-reducing aromatic oils like camphor and myrrh.
Basti (Enemas)	Enemas (Basti) work on this marma internally. Sesame oil enemas are particularly good for reducing Vata at this site. For this purpose use 1/2 cup of warm water and 1/2 cup of sesame oil as an enema and hold internally in the rectum for at least twenty minutes. This is for high Vata conditions of debility, insomnia and anxiety.
Yoga and Meditation	Meditation on the first chakra helps us control the earth element, the sense of smell and the excretory system. For this purpose one can use the seed mantra LAM for the cosmic earth element. We should assume a seated meditation posture like the lotus pose and connect with the Earth energy through the base of the spine. For both spiritual and physical health one can meditate upon the Deity Ganesha in this chakra using the mantra OM GAM Ganeshaya Namah! The yogic practice of Mulabandha, which involves tightening the muscles of the perineum, is also good for this marma.
Treatment If Injured	Injury to this marma can be traumatic. The person can become unconscious. Use herbs and oils to regain consciousness like camphor, calamus or musk, particularly as inhaled through the nose. To relieve pain, use analgesic herbs like valerian, jatamamsi, kava kava, or bayberry. Administer laxative herbs like Triphala or haritaki, if constipation is involved.

Basti marma

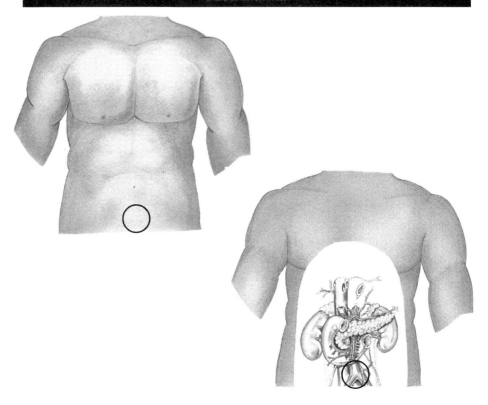

Basti

Description	
Name	Basti (bladder)
Number	1 marma point
Type	Ligament (Snayu)
Size	4 anguli (finger units)
Site	In between pubic symphisis and umbilicus in region of lower abdomen. The surrounding surface area above the bladder.
Controls	Controls the muscular system and bodily fat (Mamsavaha and Medovaha Srotamsi) and Kapha, the urinary and reproductive systems (Mutravaha and Shukravaha Srotamsi) and the second chakra (Svadishthana) and Kuhu Nali. Relates to Vata's site of accumulation in the large intestine, which is located peripheral to it, and to Apana Vayu (downward-moving air).

Anatomical Structures	Hypogastric artery, abdominal wall, external iliac and internal iliac arteries and veins. Drainage to medial sacral and internal and external iliac lymph glands. Pelvic splanchnic nerve, which supplies spleen, pancreas and hypogastric plexus. Rectus abdominus and oblique externus muscles. Pubic ligaments, median umbilical fold, superior and inferior. Symphysis pubis.
Qualities Relative to Injury	Sadya Pranahara (Immediate Death-Causing) type marma. Fiery in degree of vulnerability. Sometimes grouped under Vaikalyakara (Disability-Causing).
Symptoms If Injured	Severe injury can cause death, while even minor injuries often result in disability.

Treatment

Massage, Acupressure and Aroma Therapy	Massage gently in broad circular motions with the palm of the hand and fingers. Gentle but steady acupressure here is also good. These help reduce Vata, dispel gas and bloating, and strengthen Ojas and the reproductive system. Warm oil massage here is excellent for controlling and reducing Vata, particularly in cases of nervous exhaustion or sexual debility. Use strengthening massage oils like Dashamula Taila, Narayan Taila, plain sesame oil or castor oil. Massage slowly and gently as the region is sensitive. Use aromatic oils like nutmeg, valerian, lotus or sandalwood for calming and grounding action on Vata and for strengthening Ojas and the reproductive function. Carminative (gas-dispelling) aromas applied here like cardamom, asafoetida (hing) or basil help remove Vata or gas and distention in the large intestine. Kapha types often carry excess weight and water and have lax muscle tone in the region. They can benefit by stronger massage along with penetrating aromatic oils like cinnamon, cloves or camphor.
Yoga and Meditation	Meditation on the second chakra, which is connected to this marma, brings control of the water element, the sense of taste and the urino-genital organs. For this purpose one can use the seed mantra VAM for the cosmic water element.
Treatment If Injured	Any significant injury requires immediate medical attention. For minor injury to the bladder, Ayurveda uses a decoction of shatavari and punarnava for seven days. A good western equivalent would be marshmallow and uva ursi.

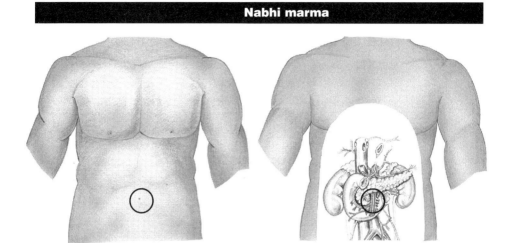

Nabhi marma

Nabhi

Description	
Name	Nabhi (navel)
Number	1 marma point
Type	Vessel (Sira)
Size	4 anguli (finger units)
Site	The navel and surrounding area, behind and around the umbilicus, so a large marma region.
Controls	Controls third or navel chakra (Manipura), Vishvodhara nadi as well as digestive, blood and circulatory systems (Annavaha and Raktavaha Srotamsi). Main pranic center for digestion and exertion. Controls Agni (digestive fire), Pachaka Pitta (digestive juices), Ranjaka Pitta (coloring of blood and bile), Samana Vayu (balancing energy), Pitta dosha and the fire element in the body as a whole.
Anatomical Structures	Inferior epigastric artery and vein. Inferior vena cava. Abdominal aorta. Solar plexus of nerves. Rectus abdominus, external and internal oblique muscles.
Qualities Relative to Injury	Sadya Pranahara (Immediate Death-Causing) type marma. Fiery in degree of vulnerability.
Symptoms If Injured	Simple injury does not cause sudden death. However if the abdominal aorta is ruptured then it can cause death from shock

and hemorrhage. Deep injury may also cause reflex stoppage of the heart.

Treatment

Massage, Acupressure and Aroma Therapy	Apply marma massage to the area, using a circular motion around the navel for about five minutes. Acupressure is done only gently since this a sensitive place. Simply laying on of the hands along with a gentle massage is often enough. A prime area for reducing Pitta and stopping its accumulation in the small intestine. Use Dashamula Taila, sesame oil or almond oil to relieve stress, nervous tension and counter nervous indigestion (Vata). For Pitta-caused heat and stress in the navel use Brahmi Taila or coconut oil. For increasing Agni (digestive power) use aromatic oils that stimulate digestion like bay, ginger, fennel or cardamom. For hyperacidity and high Pitta, massage with cooling aromatic oils like mogra (jasmine), rose or sandalwood. Clove oil is good for increasing digestive power in Pitta type people. Simply placing the hand over the navel has a protective and nurturing affect, calming Vata, particularly if the therapist has a strong power of Prana.
Herbal Paste (Lepa)	Sandalwood paste is good for alleviating Pitta (acidity) in the small intestine. A paste of asafoetida powder (hing) is good for dispelling gas and distention (Vata).
Purgation (Virechana)	Internally the use of purgative herbs like senna, rhubarb root or triphala (in large dosages) is used to remove Pitta from the navel region. It is part of Pancha Karma therapy and used only under strict clinical supervision.
Acupuncture (Suchi-karma)	For reducing fluid accumulation in the abdomen, select a point four anguli (finger units) distal to the lateral paramedian line.
Yoga and Meditation	Meditation here can help balance all the Pranas, strengthen digestion and improve physical strength. The mantra KRIM can be used here to develop energy and power of action. Meditation on the third chakra strengthens the fire element, the sense of sight, and the feet as a motor organ. For this purpose one can use the seed mantra RAM for the cosmic fire element.
Treatment If Injured	If bleeding occurs, apply cold water or ice to the area and give hemostatic herbs internally like alum, plantain or turmeric. To relieve pain, pour a continuous drip of mixture of ghee and oil over the marma area for thirty minutes.

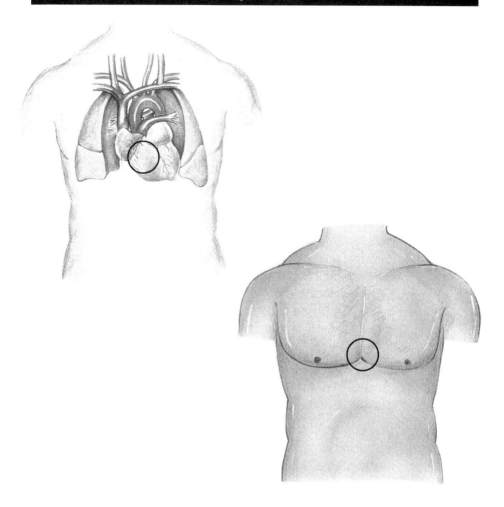

Hridaya marma

Hridaya

Description	
Name	Hridaya (heart)
Number	1 marma point
Type	Vessel (Sira)
Size	4 anguli (finger units)
Site	General region of the heart, middle of sternum, a large marma region.

Controls	Controls plasma, blood and circulatory systems (Rasavaha and Raktavaha Srotamsi), Sadhaka Pitta (power of mind), Vyana and Prana Vayus (overall powers of vitality and circulation), Ojas (strength and immunity), Tarpaka Kapha, Avalambaka Kapha (lubrication of the heart and lungs), Varuna nadi, and the fourth or heart chakra (Anahata). Also aids in the flow of breast milk. The heart is the seat of both mind (chitta) and consciousness (the higher Self or Atman). It is the region where our awareness dwells during the state of deep sleep. It governs the pranic and soul forms of Agni.
Anatomical Structures	Ascending aorta. Superior and inferior vena ceva and pulmonary veins from lungs. Drainage to tracheo-bronchial lymph glands. Vagus nerve. Cardiac muscle. Sternum bone with second, third and fourth ribs.
Qualities Relative to Injury	Sadya Pranahara (Immediate Death-Causing) type marma. Fiery in degree of vulnerability.
Symptoms If Injured	Injury will cause difficulty breathing, internal bleeding, shock and death.

Treatment

Massage, Acupressure and Aroma Therapy	Massage in a broad and gentle way using the palm of the hand. Simply placing the hand over the heart has a calming affect, particularly if the therapist has a strong power of Prana. Acupressure at the central point of the sternum can also be used to release stress and negative emotions. Sesame oil massage is good for calming the region and reducing Vata. Mustard oil is better for improving circulation and removing stagnation and Kapha. For alleviating Pitta in cases of inflammatory diseases of the heart like pericarditis, massage the heart region with Brahmi Taila, sandalwood oil, or sweet aromatic oils like jasmine, lotus, rose and saffron. Sandalwood oil will relieve both Vata and Pitta from the heart and help promote calm and sleep. Eucalyptus oil will clear Kapha from the heart. Ginger, cinnamon or elecampane aromatic oils will stimulate the circulation.

Hrid Basti (Oil Bath on the Heart)	Hrid basti, a special Ayurvedic method of bathing the heart region in sesame oil or medicated oils like Ashwagandha Taila is very effective for controlling aggravated Vata, in cases of irregular heartbeat, arrhythmia and angina pectoris. For this purpose a large amount of warm oil is used either as a drip or as held on the area (using a ring of flour dough or other substances to keep the oil from dripping away). This treatment is similar to the Shirodhara used for the head.
Yoga and Meditation	Meditation on the heart calms the mind, relieves emotional stress and helps promote deep sleep (and yoga nidra). Meditation on the heart chakra strengthens the air element, the skin, sense of touch and the hands as a motor organ. It is important for developing the inner healing powers of Prana. For this purpose one can use the seed mantra YAM for the cosmic air element or the heart mantra HRIM. Shifting one's attention from the head to the heart is also an important method of Pratyahara or internalization of the mind and senses, for overcoming anxiety and agitation. The heart is the center for the higher Self as well as for any form of God that one may worship. One can meditate upon these here.
Treatment If Injured	If there is any significant injury, immediate medical attention is required. For minor bleeding in the region, apply cold water or ice to the area and give hemostatic herbs internally like turmeric, alum or plantain. In the case of minor injuries pour a continuous drip of the mixture of ghee and sesame oil for twenty minutes. If there is difficulty breathing or reduced heart function give teas of herbs like elecampane, cinnamon, ginger or bayberry.

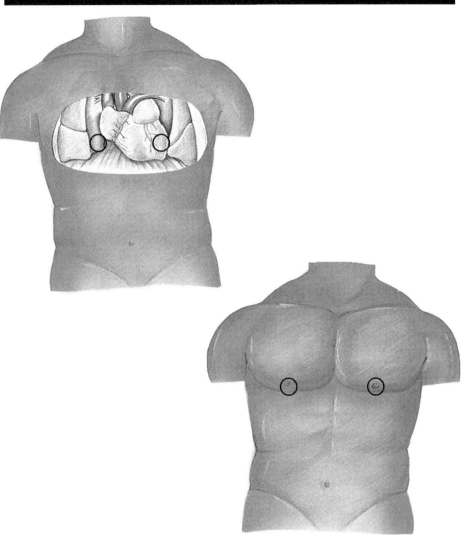

Stanamula

Description	
Name	Stanamula (root of the breast)
Number	2 marma points (one on each breast)
Type	Vessel (Sira)
Size	2 anguli (finger units)

Site	A medium-sized marma related to the nipples. Best manipulated by the point immediately below the nipples.
Controls	Controls muscular system (Mamsavaha Srotas), particularly in region of the chest, Avalambaka Kapha (lubrication to the chest), Prana and Vyana Vayus (energy circulation) and blood pressure. Governs lactation in women (Stanyavaha Srotas).
Anatomical Structures	Internal mammary artery and vein. Drainage to axillary lymph glands. Vagus nerve and intercostal nerves. Pectoralis major and minor muscles. Intercostal muscles.
Qualities Relative to Injury	Kalantara Pranahara (Long-term Death-Causing) type marma. Both fiery and watery in degree of vulnerability.
Symptoms If Injured	Deep injury can cause difficulty breathing, bleeding and eventual death.
Treatment	
Massage, Acupressure and Aroma Therapy	Massage or apply acupressure with care as this is a sensitive region. For controlling Mamsavaha Srotas (muscular system) massage with Karpas-asthyadi Taila, almond oil or sesame oil. Use aromatic oils like camphor, cinnamon, juniper, saffron or myrrh for improving circulation and reducing Kapha in the region of the heart and chest.
Treatment If Injured	If there is minor bleeding, give hemostatic herbs internally like turmeric, plantain, arjuna or nagakeshara. If there is edema, apply the paste of camphor and flaxseed.

Stanarohita marma

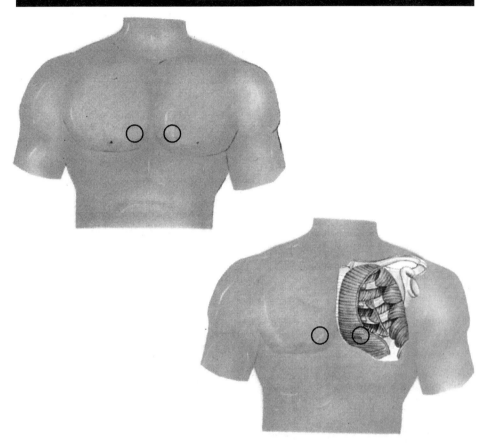

Stanarohita

Description	
Name	Stanarohita (upper region of the breast)
Number	2 marma points (one on each breast)
Type	Muscle (Mamsa)
Size	1/2 anguli (finger unit)
Site	Two anguli (finger units) directly above and to the center of the nipples (superomedial), on the edge of the muscles above the breasts.
Controls	Controls muscular and nervous systems (Mamsavaha and Majjavaha Srotamsi), Prana and Vyana Vayus, the lungs and aids in the flow of breast milk (Stanyavaha Srotas).

Anatomical Structures	Intercostal muscles, pectoralis major and minor muscles, a portion of the latissimus dorsi muscle, the fourth rib. Vagus nerve. Pulmonary and internal mammary artery and ascending aorta. Superior vena cava and internal mammary vein.
Qualities Relative to Injury	Kalantara Pranahara (Long-term Death-Causing) type marma. Both fiery and watery in degree of vulnerability.
Symptoms If Injured	Injury to the pulmonary artery will cause hemorrhage, collapse and eventual death.

Treatment

Massage, Acupressure and Aroma Therapy	Apply marma massage to the area, using a strong circular motion, for about five minutes. Acupressure works well here for calming the emotions and relieving emotional tension. The right marma connects more with the right lung, while the left marma connects more with the left lung. Use sesame oil, almond oil or Ashwagandha Taila for calming Vata and relieving anxiety. For Mamsavaha Srotas and Majjavaha Srotas (muscular and nervous systems) use aromatic oils like basil, sage, valerian, myrrh, juniper or sandalwood. For relieving cough and reducing Kapha, use aromatic oils like eucalyptus, mint or camphor, rubbing them in at this point.
Acupuncture (Suchi-karma)	For treating pleurisy and lung abscess, select a point one anguli (finger units) lateral to the areola of the breast.
Treatment If Injured	There can be bleeding or shock from injury of the blood vessels and nerves in the adjoining area. For this, use hemostatic herbs like turmeric, alum or sandalwood. Sitopaladi powder is a good Ayurvedic remedy for cough and difficult breathing after injury to this area.

Apalapa marma

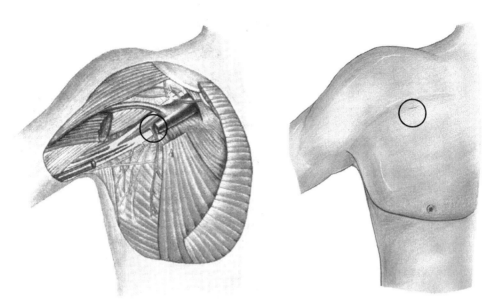

Apalapa

Description	
Name	Apala͵pa (unguarded; the armpit at the axilla)
Number	2 marma points, one on each side
Type	Vessel (Sira)
Size	1/2 anguli (finger units)
Site	In the region of the armpit, one-half anguli (finger units) lateral and downward to the center of the line joining the sternal and acromial end of the clavicle, origin of the pectoralis minor below the corocoid process, just below Kakshadhara.
Controls	Controls nervous system (Majjavaha Srotas), nerve flow to the arms, and Vyana Vayu (peripheral circulation to the arms).
Anatomical Structures	Subclavian artery and vein. Drainage to the axillary lymph glands. Brachial plexus of nerves. Pectoralis major and biceps muscles.
Qualities Relative to Injury	Kalantara Pranahara (Long-term Death-Causing) marma. Both fiery and watery in degree of vulnerability.

Symptoms If Injured	Penetrating type of injury to the subclavian artery will cause severe bleeding.
Treatment	
Massage, Acupressure and Aroma Therapy	Follow usual massage methods, using the fingers for easier access to the point. This is also a good marma for acupressure for relieving muscular and nervous tension to the shoulders, back and neck. For controlling Majjavaha Srotas (nervous system), use Asana-eladi Taila, Ashwagandha Taila, almond oil or sesame oil. Use anti-spasmodic aromatic oils like valerian, jatamamsi, lotus or basil, which relieve muscular tension.
Treatment If Injured	If there is bleeding, apply ice or hemostatic herbs like alum, turmeric or arnica. Afterwards apply an antiseptic paste made up of a mixture of triphala, milk and ghee to the injured area. Alternatively, have the patient take a tincture of myrrh or golden seal. Good Ayurvedic herbs for this condition are guggul and shilajit.

Apastambha marma

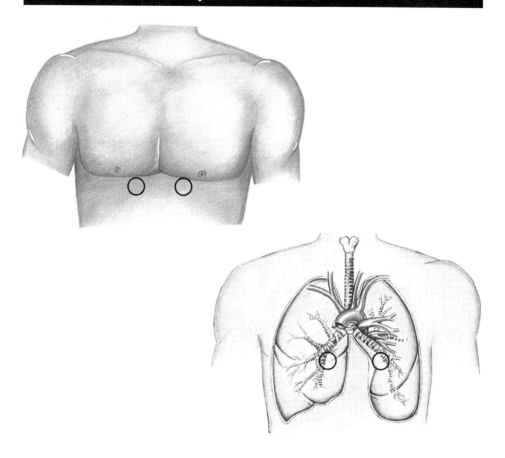

Apastambha

Description	
Name	Apastambha (standing to the side; a point on the upper abdomen said to carry Prana or life-force)
Number	2 marma points, one on each side
Type	Vessel (Sira)
Size	1/2 anguli (finger unit)
Site	Medial and downwards from the nipples at the level of the third rib immediately lateral to sternum.

Controls	Controls Kledaka Kapha (Kapha digestive juices), bone and fat tissues and channels (Asthivaha and Medovaha Srotamsi).
Anatomical	Pulmonary artery and tributaries of pulmonary vein, descending aorta. Drainage to pectoral group and trachio-bronchial as well as broncho-pulmonary lymph glands. Vagus nerve and bronchus. Pectoralis major and minor muscles and intercostal muscle.
Qualities Relative to Injury	Kalantara Pranahara (Long-term Death-Causing) type marma. Both fiery and watery in degree of vulnerability.
Symptoms If Injured	Injury to the bronchi and surrounding vessels causes bleeding that can be severe.
Treatment	
Massage, Acupressure and Aroma Therapy	Follow the usual massage procedures, working on the surrounding muscles. It is a good treatment area for reducing Kapha, preventing it from accumulating at its site in the stomach. For controlling Medovaha and Asthivaha Srotamsi (bone and fat), use Kshirabala Taila, mustard oil or sesame oil for massage. Use aromatic oils that reduce fat and heal the bones like myrrh, guggul, ginger or cinnamon. For reducing Kapha (mucus) in the lungs and treating cough, use penetrating aromatic oils like camphor, eucalyptus or myrrh. Acupressure here aids in weight reduction and controlling Kapha as well as for increasing Prana.
Treatment If Injured	Pneumonia may result from injury. Treat as per Apalapa Marma.

CHAPTER 11

Marmas on the Back and Hips

7 Regions and 14 Points

These marmas are the main points governing the hips and shoulder bones, which are the two main joints in the body. The hips are an important site of the accumulation of Kapha and fat tissue in the body. They are connected to the lymphatic system and to Ojas or primary vitality. The shoulders are an important site for Prana and strength in the body, being connected to the lungs and the heart. Points on these regions can generally take considerable pressure and strong massage, including the elbow. Various methods of back massage work well on them.

Two extra marmas can be added to these seven. Another marma can be added at the spine at the place of the navel, with points on each side of the spine 1/2 finger units in size. Treating it has the same effects as treating the navel (Nabhi marma). Another marma can be added at the spine at the place of the heart, similarly with points on each side of the spine 1/2 finger units in size. Treating it has the same effects as treating the heart (Hridaya marma). These two extra marmas that correspond to these two chakras on the back are often treated through aroma therapy and acupressure. The two, however, are not part of the classical 107 marmas.

Katikataruna marma

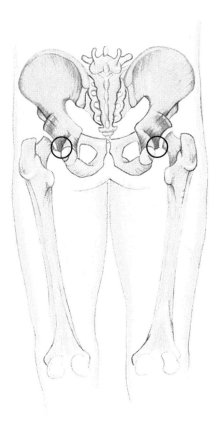 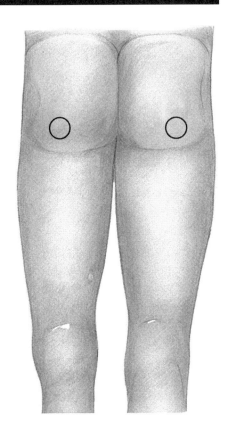

Katikataruna

Description	
Name	Katikataruna (what rises from the hip; the center of the buttocks)
Number	2 marma points, one on each side
Type	Bone (Asthi)
Size	1/2 anguli (finger unit)
Site	At the hip joint. Located two and a half anguli (finger units) downwards and inwards from the greater trochanter of the femur, the line joining the greater trochanter with the ischial tuberosity (midline between the greater trochanter and ischial tuberosity superficial to the zona orbicularis).

Controls	Controls bones and skeletal system (Asthivaha Srotas), Sleshaka Kapha (lubrication of the joints) and Swedavaha Srotas (sweat glands). Relieves Vata.
Anatomical Structures	Posterior aspect of ileum, sacroiliac ligaments. Superior gluteal artery and vein. Drainage of common iliac lymph glands. Sacral plexus of nerves. Gluteus maximus muscle.
Qualities Relative to Injury	Kalantara Pranahara (Long-term Death-Causing) type marma. Both fiery and watery in degree of vulnerability.
Symptoms If Injured	Injury to the artery will lead to hemorrhage and anemia.

Treatment	
Massage, Acupressure and Aroma Therapy	Apply marma massage to the area, using a strong circular motion for about five minutes. Strong acupressure can also be done at this point for relieving tension in the hips and pelvis (the elbow can be used for more force if necessary). For controlling Asthivaha Srotas (bones) and Sleshaka Kapha, use Dhanvantara Taila, Gandha Taila, Bhringaraj Taila, Ashwagandha Taila, almond oil or sesame oil. Use aromatic oils which heal the bones like myrrh, guggul, camphor or wintergreen. For controlling Swedavaha Srotas (sweating system) use Kakolyadi Taila or mustard oil for massage. Use sweat-promoting aromatic oils like camphor, eucalyptus, mint or sage.
Acupuncture (Suchi-karma)	For treating old fevers or remittent fevers, select a point at the center of sacral joint for acupuncture.
Treatment If Injured	Apply a bandage for relieving pain and stopping bleeding. Apply a paste of turmeric, sandalwood and licorice on the injured area.

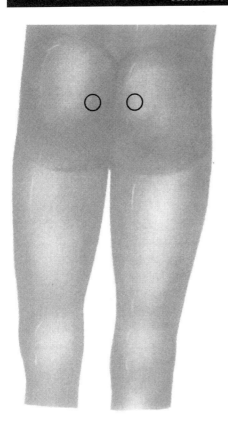
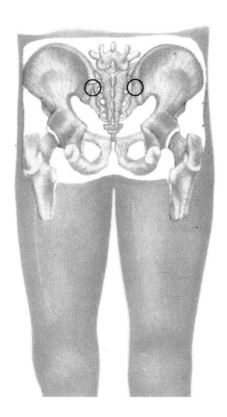

Kukundara marma

Kukundara

Description	
Name	Kukundara (on the loins on either side of posterior superior iliac spine)
Number	2 marma points, one on each side of the back
Type	Joint (Sandhi)
Size	1/2 anguli (finger unit)
Site	On both posterior superior iliac spine notches, just above buttocks (inside or spinal area of the hip bone).

Controls	Controls circulatory system and blood formation (Raktavaha Srotas and formation of Rakta Dhatu) and Ranjaka Pitta (coloring of the blood) as well as the menstrual system. Also relates to the second or sex chakra (Svadhishtana), Ojas and Apana Vayu.
Anatomical Structures	Ilium bone. Ischium bone (no joint structure). Inferior gluteal artery and vein. Inferior pudendal artery and vein. Sciatic nerve. Gluteus maximus and levator ani muscles.
Qualities Relative to Injury	Vaikalyakara (Disability-Causing) type marma. Watery in degree of vulnerability.
Symptoms If Injured	Injury to the sciatic nerve will lead to loss of sensation and paralysis of the lower limb.

Treatment

Massage, Acupressure and Aroma Therapy	Apply marma massage to the area, using a strong circular motion for about five minutes. Strong acupressure can also be applied here. For stimulating Raktavaha Srotas (blood and circulatory system) use Manjishtadi Taila or Kottamchukadi (calamus, garlic and galangal) Taila or massage oils like safflower and mustard. Use aromatic oils that stimulate blood flow like angelica, saffron, rosemary, turmeric or myrrh. Massage the area with tonifying oils like Shatavari Taila or Ashwagandha Taila or plain sesame oil for weakness of the blood.
Yoga and Meditation	Meditation on the second chakra, which is connected to this marma, brings control of the water element, the sense of taste and the urino-genital organs. For this purpose one can use the seed mantra VAM for the cosmic water element.
Treatment If Injured	Apply a warm sesame oil drip (dhara) on the marma area. To remove pain and edema use a paste of sandalwood, turmeric and alum.

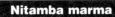

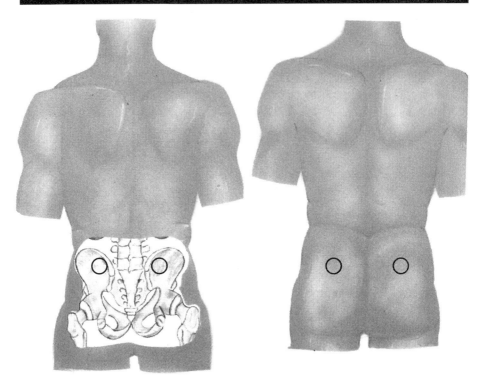

Nitamba

Description	
Name	Nitamba (upper region of the buttocks)
Number	2 marma points, one on each buttock
Type	Bone (Asthi)
Size	1/2 anguli (finger unit)
Site	One anguli (finger unit) above Kukundara marma.
Controls	Controls plasma and lymphatic system, bodily fat, skeletal system and urinary system (Rasavaha, Medovaha, Asthivaha and Mutravaha Srotamsi) as well as the kidneys: an important Kapha point.

Anatomical Structures	Ilium and sacrum bone, sacroiliac joint, anterior and posterior. Sacroiliac ligaments. Sacral plexus of nerves. Psoas major and iliac muscles.
Qualities Relative to Injury	Kalantara Pranahara (Long-term Death-Causing) type of marma. Both fiery and watery in degree of vulnerability.
Symptoms If Injured	Injury to the iliac bone and sacral plexus will cause functional loss and wasting of the muscles.

Treatment

Massage, Acupressure and Aroma Therapy	Apply marma massage to the area, using a strong circular motion for about five minutes. Strong acupressure here aids in weight reduction and in controlling Kapha. The elbows can be used for more force if necessary. For controlling Rasavaha Srotas (lymphatic system) massage with Nimba Taila or mustard oil, along with stimulating aromatic oils like camphor or cardamom. For controlling Asthivaha Srotas (skeletal system) massage with Nimbapatradi Taila or sesame oil and analgesic aromatic oils like myrrh, guggul, valerian or wintergreen.
Treatment If Injured	For edema, apply a paste of lemongrass and shatavari (or horsetail). Later on, massage with Shatavari Taila. An anuvasana or oil enema may be helpful.

Parshvasandhi marma

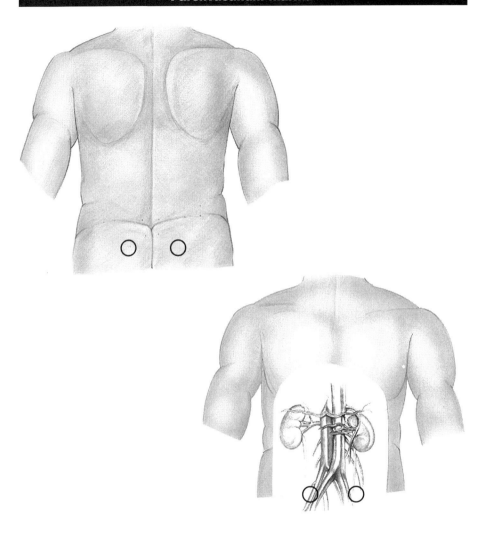

Parshvasandhi

Description	
Name	Parshvasandhi (the side of the waist)
Number	2 marma points
Type	Vessel (Sira)
Size	1/2 anguli (finger unit)
Site	The location on posterior side is the lateral aspect of the

	lumbosacral joint. But on the anterior side, the marma point is close to the common iliac artery.
Controls	Controls the second chakra (Svadhishthana), adrenal glands, ovaries and the channels of digestive, excretory and respiratory systems (Annavaha, Purishavaha and Pranahava Srotamsi). Connects to the power of Ojas, which manifests through the legs.
Anatomical Structures	Common iliac artery and drainage of veins from pelvic and leg area. Drainage to common iliac group of lymph glands. Hypogastric plexus of nerves. Fifth lumbar and first sacral vertebrae. Lumbosacral joint.
Qualities Relative to Injury	Kalantara Pranahara (Long-term Death-Causing) type marma. Both fiery and watery in degree of vulnerability.
Symptoms If Injured	Injury to the common iliac artery will cause severe bleeding.

Treatment

Massage, Acupressure and Aroma Therapy	Follow usual massage methods, using some force and power of movement. Acupressure here strengthens Ojas, immune response and the reproductive system. Treating of this marma goes along well with treating Basti and Vitapa marmas on the other side of the body. For controlling the second chakra (Svadhishthana), adrenal and ovaries, massage with Vacha-lashunadi Taila or with sesame oil. Use aromatic oils like nutmeg, pennyroyal, musk or saffron. Use Bala Taila or Ashwagandha Taila for general strengthening purposes.
Acupuncture (Suchi-karma)	For treating dysentery and diarrhea select a point 4 anguli (finger units) medial to the marma.
Treatment If Injured	If there is bleeding after injury, apply a bandage and give hemostatic herbs internally like turmeric and alum. Give complete bed rest to the patient.

Brihati marma

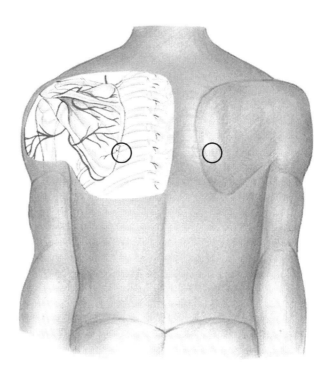

Brihati

Description	
Name	Brihati (the large or the broad region of the back)
Number	2 marma points (one on each side of the back)
Type	Vessel (Sira)
Size	1/2 anguli (finger units)
Site	Between the shoulder blades, three anguli (finger units) above the inferior angle of the scapula on the inner edge, at the triangular space.

Controls	Controls the third or navel chakra (Manipura), Pitta and Tejas (courage and valor that manifests through the arms), Swedavaha Srotas (sweating), Bhrajaka Pitta (heat absorption on the skin), Vyana Vayu, and plasma and lymphatic system (Rasavaha Srotas).
Anatomical Structures	Subscapular artery and vein. Drainage to the subscapular group of axillary lymph glands. Suprascapular and circumflex nerve. Infra spinatus, tres major and minor, and trapezius muscles.
Qualities Relative to Injury	Kalantara Pranahara (Long-term Death-Causing) type marma. Both fiery and watery in degree of vulnerability.
Symptoms If Injured	Superficial injury will cause damage to the vessels and deep injury will cause damage to the lungs.

Treatment

Massage, Acupressure and Aroma Therapy	Apply marma massage to the area, using a strong circular motion for about five minutes. Acupressure here can relieve tension and stress in the shoulders, back and heart. Treatment of this marma often combines well with that of Hridaya marma on the opposite side of the body. For improving the functions of Rasavaha Srotas (plasma and lymphatic system), use Rasa Taila, Himasagara Taila or mustard oil and stimulating aromatic oils like cardamom, camphor or eucalyptus.
Acupuncture (Suchi-karma)	For treating a frozen shoulder or atrophy of the arm muscles, select a point one anguli (finger unit) medial to the marma.
Treatment If Injured	This is a vessel (Sira) marma and so bleeds easily. For bleeding apply ice, take hemostatic herbs and give complete bed rest to the patient. A mild laxative like triphala can be helpful.

Amsaphalaka marma

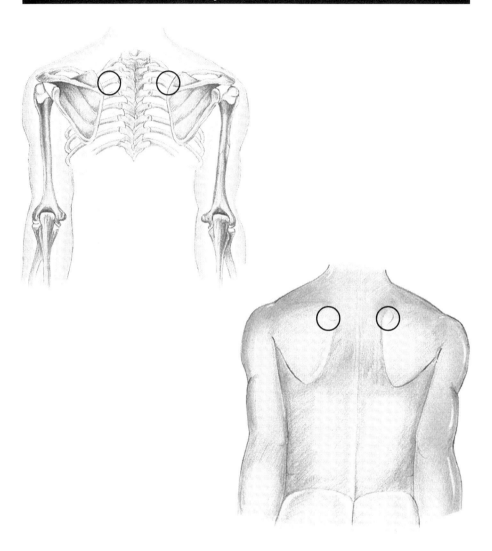

Amsaphalaka

Description	
Name	Amsaphalaka (shoulder blade)
Number	2 marma points (one on each shoulder-blade)
Type	Bone (Asthi)
Size	1/2 anguli (finger unit)

Site	On the scapula bone above Brihati, superomedial angle of the scapula.
Controls	Controls respiratory system (Pranavaha Srotas), Sleshaka Kapha (lubrication of the joints), Prana and Vyana Vayus (energy circulation) and fourth or heart chakra (Anahata).
Anatomical Structures	Fifth, sixth, seventh cervical and first thoracic vertebrae. Subclavian artery and vein. Fifth, sixth and seventh thoracic nerves. Trapezius and major rhomboid muscles.
Qualities Relative to Injury	Vaikalyakara (Disability-Causing) type marma. Watery in degree of vulnerability.
Symptoms If Injured	Injury to the nerve may cause dysfunction of the muscles, leading to disability and wasting away of the muscle tissue.

Treatment

Massage, Acupressure and Aroma Therapy	Apply marma massage to the area, using a strong circular motion for about five minutes. Acupressure here helps open the Prana in the arms, lungs and chest, improving the function of Vyana (peripheral circulation). For improving the functions of Pranavaha Srotas (respiratory system), use Mahanarayan Taila, Shefali Taila, almond oil or sesame oil. Use stimulating aromatic oils like eucalyptus, mint or camphor which open up the lungs and chest.
Treatment If Injured	For relieving edema and pain apply paste of sandalwood and khus (if available, otherwise sandalwood by itself is fine). Later on massage the area with anti-Vata oils like Dashamula Taila, Bala Taila or sesame oil. If there is a fracture, apply a bandage and give rest to the part.

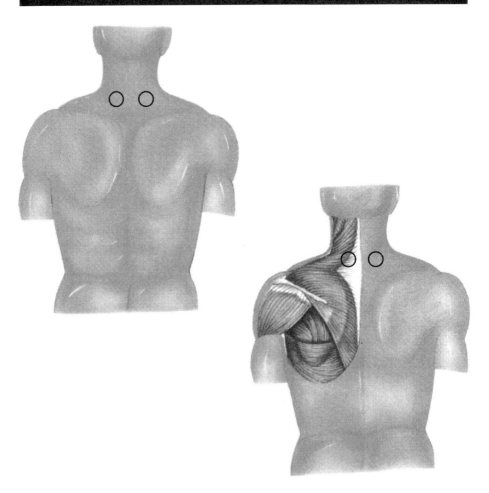

Amsa marma

Amsa

Description	
Name	Amsa (shoulder)
Number	2 marma points (one on each shoulder)
Type	Ligament (Snayu)
Size	1/2 anguli (finger unit)
Site	Between the neck and arms, on the trapezius muscle, one half-anguli (finger unit) lateral to the spinous process of the fifth cervical vertebra.

Controls	Controls the fifth or throat chakra (Vishuddha), Bhrajaka Pitta (heat absorption on the skin), Udana Vayu (upward movement of Prana) and the brain.
Anatomical Structures	Trapezius and levator scapuli muscles. Subscapular artery and vein. Drainage to the subscapular group of axillary glands. Scapula bone and coracoacromial and suprascapular ligaments. Phrenic, third and fourth cervical nerves.
Qualities Relative to Injury	Vaikalyakara (Disability-Causing) type of marma. Watery in degree of vulnerability.
Symptoms If Injured	Injury to the muscles and the ligaments will result in disability.

Treatment

Massage, Acupressure and Aroma Therapy	Follow usual massage procedures, using some degree of force in the region, particularly with the thumbs. Acupressure is great here for removing tension in the neck and strengthening Udana (upward movement of energy). For controlling Bhrajaka Pitta (Pitta in the skin), massage with Brahmi Taila or with sunflower or coconut oils. Use aromatic oils like jasmine, sandalwood, wormwood or chamomile. For Udana Vayu, aromatic oils that work on the throat are good like bayberry, mint or sage.
Yoga and Meditation	Meditation on the fifth or throat chakra gives control over the ether element, the sense quality of sound, the ears and speech. For this purpose one can use the seed mantra HAM for the cosmic ether element. Meditation here gives control over all the senses and elements through the element of ether and the sense quality of sound. The mantra AIM, which gives power over speech, works well here. Also good for concentration to improve the dream state, as the soul is said to dwell in the throat while dream.
Treatment If Injured	The same as Amsaphalaka.

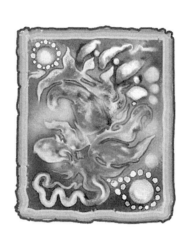

CHAPTER 12

Marmas on the Head and Neck

14 Regions and 37 points

The head and neck, with their sensitive regions, sensory openings and connection to the brain, have the largest number of marmas. The head is where we have our greatest reception of both Prana and nutrients through the senses, nose and mouth. The neck determines our posture and blood flow to the head. Proper alignment of the upper back, neck and head is crucial for clarity of mind and the practice of meditation. Marmas on the head are important for treating psychological conditions and nervous system disorders.

Marmas on the head are often more easily treated through acupressure than through massage as they are usually small in size. Application of heavy oils to the head such as sesame are very calming, settling the nerves and inducing sleep. Spicy aromatic oils to the head like eucalyptus or ginger are good for clearing the sinuses and stimulating the mind and senses. The marmas on the face and head are particularly good for acupressure and facial massage. The marmas on the top of the head can be treated through massage of the skull.

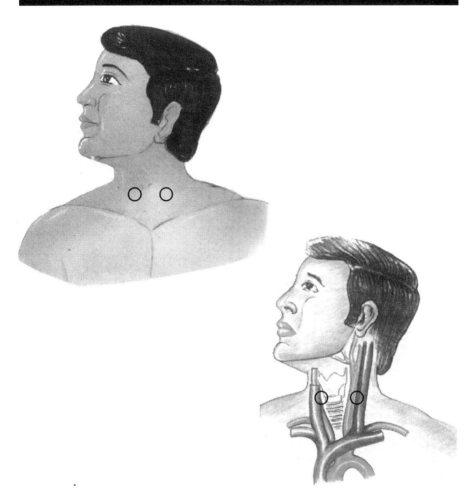

Nila

Description	
Name	Nila (dark blue, the color of the veins at this point)
Number	2 marma points (one on each side of the neck)
Type	Vessel (Sira)
Size	4 anguli (finger units)
Site	A large area of the lower neck, with the main points just lateral to the trachea. The main vulnerable site is the trachea itself. One can also feel the pulse at this location.

Controls	Controls Bhrajaka Pitta (heat absorption of the skin), Udana Vayu (upward-moving Prana), speech, thyroid and circulation to the brain.
Anatomical Structures	This marma is located on the internal jugular vein. Upper deep cervical group of lymph glands. Accessory nerves supplying sternomastoid and recurrent laryngeal branch. Primary rami of the fourth, fifth and sixth cervical nerves.
Qualities Relative to Injury	Vaikalyakara (Disability-Causing) type marma. Watery in degree of vulnerability.
Symptoms If Injured	Although the name Nila indicates blood vessels, the symptoms are of injury to the vocal cords leading to loss of voice.

Treatment

Massage, Acupressure and Aroma Therapy	Massage only very lightly as the neck is a sensitive region. Oil application is more important than applying pressure. A gentle touch to convey Prana is all that is required. Acupressure is usually not performed on this marma. For Bhrajaka Pitta (Pitta in the skin) use Brahmi Taila, Bhringaraj Taila or plain coconut oil. Use cooling aromatic oils like sandalwood, chamomile, cloves, coriander, rose or wormwood. For improving the voice use aromatic oils of calamus, bayberry or peppermint that open the throat. These can also help in the case of sore throat, laryngitis or similar difficulties.
Yoga and Meditation	A good place for concentration and meditation to improve the voice and the power of speech, increasing Prana and circulation to the throat. Use the mantra AIM (sacred to Sarasvati, the Goddess of Speech) for this purpose. For strengthening throat chakra, one can use the seed mantra HAM for controlling the cosmic ether element. Also good for concentration to improve the dream state, as the soul is said to dwell in the throat while dreaming.
Treatment If Injured	The patient may develop loss of speech or loss of the sensation of taste. For this take calamus, licorice and ginger along with honey as a powder or tea. Similarly, this being a vessel marma inury may cause bleeding. As a sensitive region it is best to seek medical attention if this is the case.

Manya marma

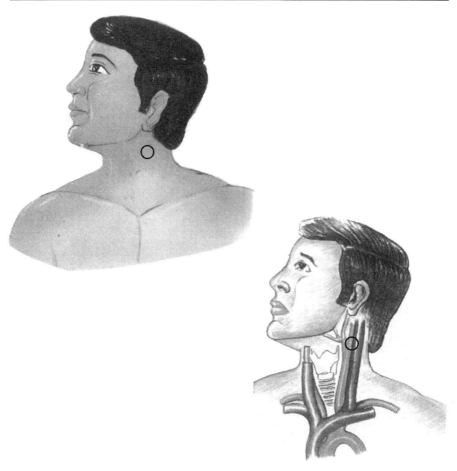

Manya

Description	
Name	Manya (honor; due to its connection with the voice)
Number	2 marma points (one on each side of the neck)
Type	Vessel (Sira)
Size	4 anguli (finger units)
Site	A large area of the middle neck, with the main point located one-half anguli (finger unit) down and back (behind) from the

	angle of mandibular bone (one-half unit inferior and one-half unit posterior to the mandibular angle).
Controls	Controls plasma, blood and circulatory system (Rasavaha and Raktavaha Srotamsi), Bodhaka Kapha (lubrication to the mouth and throat and sense of taste) and Udana Vayu (upward-moving air). A Kapha marma connected to the tongue and to salivation.
Anatomical Structures	External carotid artery, anterior jugular vein. Lymph drainage of upper cervical glands. Glassopharyngeal nerve, lingual nerve and accessory nerves.
Qualities Relative to Injury	Vaikalyakara (Disability-Causing) type marma. Watery in degree of vulnerability.
Symptoms	Injury to the nerves will result in loss of sensation and taste in the tongue or its paralysis.
Treatment	
Massage, Acupressure and Aroma Therapy	Massage or use acupressure emphasizing the point up and back to the mandibular bone, taking care to avoid pressure to the soft and sensitive tissue of the front of the neck. Aroma therapy works well here, with the oils penetrating easily into the region of the throat. For controlling Rasavaha and Raktavaha Srotamsi (circulatory system and lymphatics) and Bodhaka Kapha (lubrication of the mouth), use stimulating aromatic oils like cinnamon, cardamom, rosemary, mint or tea tree. These oils are also good for sore throat or swollen glands in the region and can help treat or prevent colds, flu and other upper respiratory problems.
Treatment If Injured	The same as Nila.

Sira Matrika marma

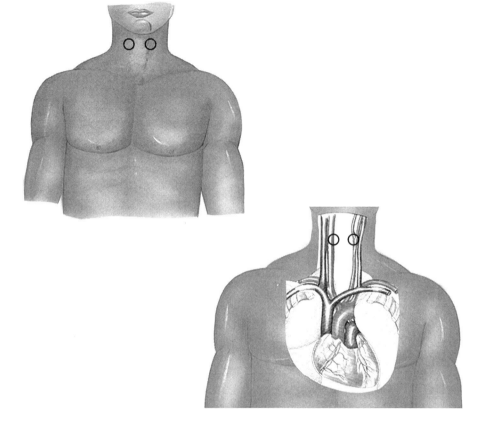

Sira Matrika

Description	
Name	Sira Matrika (mother of the blood vessels)
Number	8 marmas (4 on each side of the neck). As they are all close together, the marma is often treated as one overall region.
Type	Vessel (Sira)
Size	4 anguli (finger units)
Site	An internal marma consisting mainly of blood vessels, one-half anguli (finger unit) lateral to the outside of the trachea, situated on the different branches of the common carotid artery, a large area of the neck.

Controls	Controls blood (Raktavaha Srotas) flow from the heart to the head, Udana Vayu (upward-moving Prana), and the nervous system (Majjavaha Srotas). The main vulnerable region is the carotid artery and jugular vein. A pulse can be felt at this point, just as at nearby Nila marma.
Anatomical Structures	Branches of common carotid artery, front and back of neck, face, side of head, meninges, middle ear, thyroid, tongue, tonsils, internal ear and forehead. Internal jugular vein receiving from the face, neck and thyroid. Vagus and phrenic nerves.
Qualities Relative to Injury	Sadya Pranahara (Immediate Death-Causing) type marma. Fiery in degree of vulnerability.
Symptoms If Injured	Injury to the blood vessels will cause severe hemorrhage, collapse and death.
Treatment	
Massage, Acupressure and Aroma Therapy	Massage only very lightly as the neck is a sensitive region. Oil application is more important than applying pressure. A gentle touch to convey Prana is all that is required. Acupressure is usually not done here. Use Jyotishmati, Shankhapushpi or Ashwagandha Tailas or plain oils like almond and sesame oil for nourishing the nerves, as well as nervine aromatic oils like angelica, calamus, valerian or jatamamsi for calmative purposes. For improving blood-flow use aromatic oils like cinnamon, saffron, rosemary or myrrh. Calamus is good specifically for aiding in blood flow to the head. As with Nila marma, for improving the voice use aromatic oils of calamus, bayberry or peppermint that open the throat.
Treatment If Injured	Apply a paste of licorice and ghee to the tongue for soothing the throat. If injury is severe, seek immediate medical attention.

Phana marma

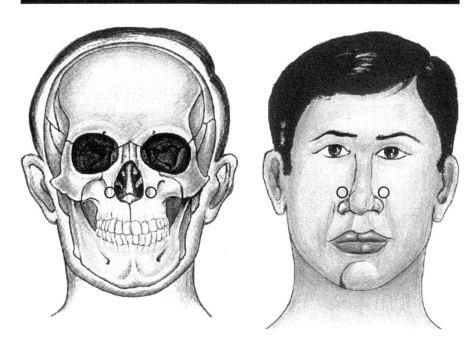

Phana

Description	
Name	Phana (a serpent's hood; on the side of nostrils)
Number	2 marma points (one on each nostril)
Type	Vessel (Sira)
Size	1/2 anguli (finger unit)
Site	The point outside at the base of the nose and the nostril openings. However, additional points exist along the side of the nose along the outside surface of the nasal bone.
Controls	Controls Prana, the sense organ of smell, Kapha in the head, the nasal passages and sinuses and the Ida and Pingala nadis (left and right nostril Prana channels).
Anatomical Structures	Facial artery and vein. Branches of olfactory nerves and facial nerve. Orbicularis oris and levator labii superior muscles. Nasal, frontal and ethmoid bones. Submandibular lymph supply.

Qualities Relative to Injury	Vaikalyakara (Disability-Causing) type marma. Watery in degree of vulnerability.
Symptoms If Injured	Injury will produce impairment of the nose and face. If the nerves are injured it may cause loss of sensation of smell.

Treatment

Massage, Acupressure and Aroma Therapy	Apply marma massage to the area, using a strong circular motion, for about five minutes. One can also massage the entire side of the nasal bone. One can massage both sides of the nose at once. This is also a good marma for acupressure, particularly using the index finger, for relieving headache, pressure in the sinuses and congestion (Kapha). Helps remove Kapha upward and outward from the lungs and sinuses. For treating the nose, spicy aromatic oils are great. Application of camphor, eucalyptus or peppermint oil to Phana marma opens the sinuses, stimulates the senses and helps relieve headaches. For massage oils, expectorant oils like mustard oil or apricot oil are good.
Nasya (Nasal Therapy)	Ayurvedic Nasya therapy (nasal therapy) is excellent for working on this marma. Special Ayurvedic medicated nasya (nasal) oils can be put in the nostrils using an eye-dropper or rubbed in with the little finger. Herbal powders like calamus or ginger can be snuffed through the nostrils in order to clear the head. For Vata and Kapha doshas and for clearing the head and sinuses, calamus (Vacha) based nasya oils are best, such as Vacha Taila. For Pitta dosha and for soothing the nostrils, licorice based oils can be used like Anu Taila. Many Ayurvedic clinics and pharmacies have their own special Nasya oils that can be purchased.
Neti Pot	The use of the Neti pot, a special yogic water pot, for pouring salt water through the nostrils helps this marma indirectly by working on its internal counterparts. It is good for conditions of dryness or congestion and for general cleansing purposes.
Acupuncture (Suchi-karma)	For treating anosmia (lack of smell) select a point 1/2 anguli (finger units) medial to this marma.

Yoga and Meditation	Phana is perhaps the most important marma for Pranayama and for the control of the Prana, particularly through the practice of alternate nostril breathing. Stimulating the right Phana marma helps open the solar or Pingala nadi. Stimulating the left Phana marma helps open the lunar or Ida nadi. Like its name as the serpent's hood, Phana marma helps energize the deeper serpent or bioelectrical force of Prana. Meditation on Prana at these two points (right and left nostrils) helps balance the flow of energy between the right and left sides of the body.
Treatment If Injured	If there is bleeding, apply ice and give a nasya (nasal application) of turmeric. Give hemostatic (stopping-bleeding) herbs like turmeric or plantain internally. For relieving pain, use a (nasal application) of Chandanadi Taila (the medicated oil, not the aromatic oil), Anu Taila or sesame oil.

Apanga marma

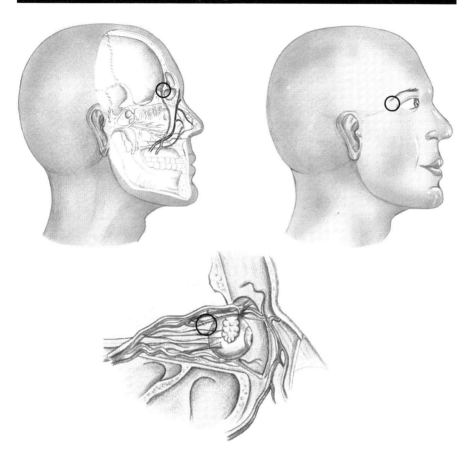

Apanga

Description	
Name	Apanga (the outer corner of the eyes)
Number	2 marma points (one by each eye)
Type	Vessel (Sira)
Size	1/2 anguli (finger unit)
Site	At the outer angle of eye, lateral side of orbital fossa, immediately posterior to the zygomatic bone level with the eye.
Controls	Controls sense organ of sight, Alochaka Pitta, and Pusha and Gandhari nadis (right and left eye channels).

Anatomical Structures	Anterior ciliary arteries and veins. Drainage to the superficial parotid lymph glands. Optic and ciliary nerves. Sphenoid, maxillary and zygomatic joints.
Qualities Relative to Injury	Vaikalyakara (Disability-Causing) type marma. Watery in degree of vulnerability.
Symptoms If Injured	Injury may produce blindness and damage to the face.

Treatment

Massage, Acupressure and Aroma Therapy	Apply marma massage to the area, using a strong circular motion for about five minutes. This is also a good marma for acupressure for photophobic headaches, clearing the upper sinuses and reducing Pitta. For treating the eyes at this point, use cooling massage oils like Brahmi Taila, Triphala ghee or plain ghee. Use cooling aromatic oils like sandalwood, khus (vetiver), or rose. But make sure not to get any aromatic oils into the eyes as this will cause irritation.
Acupuncture (Suchi-karma)	For glaucoma, headache or stye, acupuncture should be done at a point one anguli (finger unit) above this marma.
Yoga and Meditation	Meditation on the right eye is said to increase awareness and clarity of thought during the waking state. Meditation on this point or acupressure here helps control the sense organ of the eyes.
Treatment If Injured	For relieving pain in the eyes, administer a netra basti (eye wash) with ghee or Triphala ghee. Apply a paste of triphala and licorice on the marma.

Vidhura marma

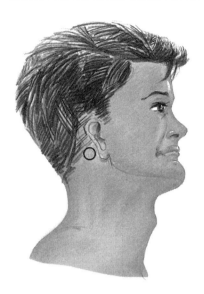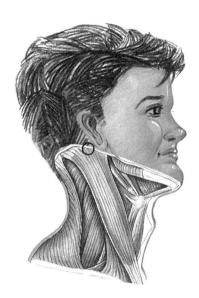

Vidhura

Description	
Name	Vidhura (distress; due to its sensitive nature)
Number	2 marma points (one by each ear)
Type	Ligament (Snayu)
Size	1/2 anguli (finger unit)
Site	Behind and below the ear, just below the mastoid bone, inferior to the tip of the mastoid process.
Controls	Controls sense organ of hearing, Prana Vayu, and Payasvini and Shankhini nadis (right and left side ear channels).
Anatomical Structures	Mastoid muscle. Facial nerve, great auricular nerve and auditory nerve. Basilar and posterior auricular arteries, posterior auricular vein.
Qualities Relative to Injury	Vaikalyakara (Disability-Causing) type marma. Watery in degree of vulnerability.

Symptoms If Injured	Injury can cause deafness.
Treatment	
Massage, Acupressure and Aroma Therapy	Follow usual massage procedures using the fingers, particularly the middle finger. Acupressure is good here for reducing Vata (anxiety and mental agitation) and clearing congestion from the ears. For treating the ears, use Dhanvantara Taila, sesame oil or almond oil for massage purposes. For decongesting the ear canal, apply penetrating aromatic oils like camphor, mint or eucalyptus.
Acupuncture (Suchi-karma)	For treating ear diseases like otalgia, carry out acupuncture 4 anguli (finger units) above this marma
Yoga and Meditation	Stimulating this point helps one hear the inner sounds (nada), particularly the right Vidhura marma. The use of acupressure or calming aromatic oils like sandalwood is good for Pratyahara of the ears (calming and controlling the sense of hearing). This is good for treating ringing in the ears and hypersensitivity to sounds.
Treatment If Injured	To relieve pain in the ear, put warm (not hot) sesame oil in the ear.

Krikatika marma

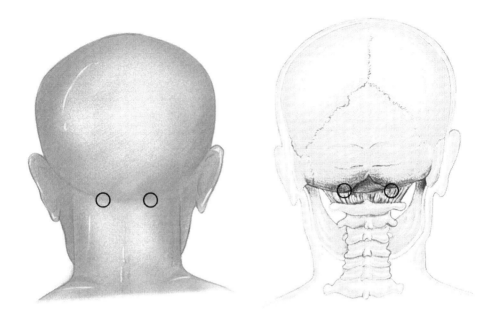

Krikatika

Description	
Name	Krikatika (the joint of the neck)
Number	2 marma points (one on each side of the neck)
Type	Joint (Sandhi)
Size	1/2 anguli (finger unit)
Site	At the junction of the neck and the head, immediately inferior to the external occipital protuberance.
Controls	Controls the bodily posture, circulation to the head, Tarpaka Kapha (contentment and lubrication to the brain) and Udana Vayu (upward-moving air that allows us to keep our back and neck straight), as well as the subconscious mind.

Anatomical Structures	Atlanto-occipital joint. Occiput and first cervical bone. Anterior longitudinal, anterior and posterior primary ramus nerves. Vertebral artery and vein. Rectus capitis lateralis and rectus capitis anterior muscles.
Qualities Relative to Injury	Vaikalyakara (Disability-Causing) type of marma. Watery in degree of vulnerability. Alternatively, Sadya Pranahara (Immediate Death-Causing) type, if injury is severe.
Symptoms If Injured	Injury to the joint will lead to limitation of the movement of the head. The dislocation of the joint can cause death by pressing on the medulla oblongata.
Treatment	
Massage, Acupressure and Aroma Therapy	Massage firmly, keeping the head balanced in the process. This is also a good point for applying strong acupressure to relieve muscular tension. For improving the posture, massage the marma area with Devadarvyadi Taila (medicated cedar oil) or with sesame oil. For congestion in the neck and sinuses use penetrating aromatic oils like bayberry, mint, eucalyptus or ginger.
Yoga and Meditation	A good point of focus for meditation to control the subconscious mind, instincts and deep-seated emotions, to aid in internalization of the mind and Pratyahara. Also relates to the third eye chakra.
Treatment If Injured	If the patient develops tremors to the head, use cedar oil or myrrh oil for massage or acupressure.

Shankha marma

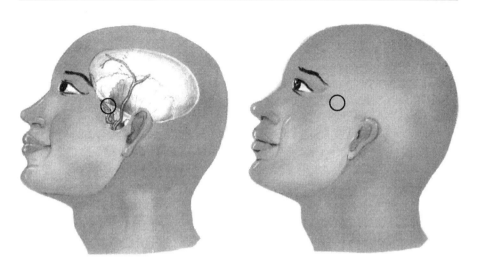

Shankha

Description	
Name	Shankha (conch; the temple)
Number	2 marma points (one on each temple)
Type	Bone (Asthi)
Size	1/2 anguli (finger unit)
Site	The temple, in between the tragus of the ear and the lateral corner of the eye (anterior aspect of temporal fossa along the junction with the sphenoid bone).
Controls	Controls sense organ of touch, Apana Vayu (downward-moving air) and Vata in the large intestine.
Anatomical Structures	Temporal bone along with temporal muscle. Temporal and internal carotid artery, temporal vein. Drainage to the superficial parotid glands. Facial and corda typmani nerves.
Qualities Relative to Injury	Sadya Pranahara (Immediate Death-Causing) type marma. Fiery in degree of vulnerability.

Symptoms If Injured	Injury may damage the brain, causing hemorrhage and possible death.
Treatment	
Massage, Acupressure and Aroma Therapy	Apply marma massage to the area, using a gentle circular motion for about five minutes. This is also a good marma for acupressure but of a gentle nature and can be used for directing energy to the brain and mind. For this, place the middle finger of one hand on one of the two Shankha marmas and the middle finger of the other hand on the other. For treating any problems of the skin or for high Vata use Ashwagandha Taila, almond oil or sesame oil. Sesame oil applied here is very calming and helps promote sleep. For headaches in the area use stimulating aromatic oils or pastes of ginger, calamus, angelica or mustard.
Acupuncture (Suchi-karma)	For treating epilepsy carry out acupuncture at the point two angulis (finger units) distal to temporo-mandibular joint.
Treatment If Injured	Injury can result in loss of consciousness. For this have the patient snuff the power of calamus or ginger to regain awareness or give Hemagarbha Taila with ginger. Give herbal teas of awareness-promoting herbs like calamus, gotu kola, brahmi, bayberry or shankhapushpi.

Utkshepa marma

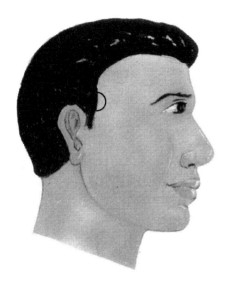
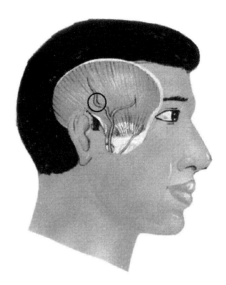

Utkshepa

Description	
Name	Utkshepa (what is cast upwards; owing to its location above the ears)
Number	2 marma points
Type	Ligament (Snayu)
Size	1/2 anguli (finger units)
Site	Behind the upper border of the helix of the ear, two anguli (finger units) above Shankha marma.
Controls	An important control point for Vata and the mind, for Apana Vayu, the large intestine and the sense organ of smell.
Anatomical Structures	Temporal muscle and bone. Temporal, zygomatic temporal and internal carotid arteries. Anterior temporal diploic vein. Second and third cervical nerves.

Qualities Relative to Injury	Vishalyaghna (Fatal If Pierced) type marma. Airy in degree of vulnerability.
Symptoms If Injured	Injury will cause bleeding, damage to the head, and cause Prana (Vata) to be quickly lost.

Treatment

Massage, Acupressure and Aroma Therapy	Follow usual massage procedures, but gently using the fingers or the thumb. Acupressure here helps calm the mind and controls Vata. For Vata disorders, use strengthening massage oils like Bala Taila, Ashwagandha Taila, sesame oil or almond oil. Use calming aromatic oils like sandalwood, basil, jatamamsi or valerian.
Acupuncture (Suchi-karma)	For treating psychological disorders and mental agitation, select a point one anguli (finger unit) above, on the border of hairline.
Treatment If Injured	The same as Shankha marma.

Avarta marma

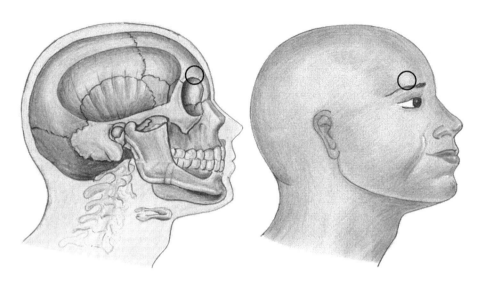

Avarta

Description	
Name	Avarta (calamity; as it is very sensitive)
Number	2 marma points (near each eye)
Type	Joint (Sandhi)
Size	1/2 anguli (finger unit)
Site	In the upper border of the orbital cavity formed by the frontal bone. At the center of each eyebrow at the base of the forehead (supraorbital notch of the frontal bone).
Controls	Controls Vata in general, Prana, the sense of sight (Alochaka Pitta) and bodily posture.
Anatomical Structures	Frontal bone, sphenoid and frontal joints. Levator superior and superior rectus muscles. Optic and frontal nerves. Ophthalmic and supraorbital arteries, superior ophthalmic vein.
Qualities Relative to Injury	Vaikalyakara (Disability-Causing) type marma. Watery in degree of vulnerability.

Symptoms If Injured	Injury will cause impairment of the face, headaches and disorientation.
Treatment	
Massage, Acupressure and Aroma Therapy	Massage gently using the fingers, particularly the middle finger. This is also a good marma for acupressure using aromatic oils, particularly for reducing high Vata. Again, be careful not to get any aromatic oils into the eye where they can cause irritation. For controlling Prana Vayu (improving energy, adaptability and equilibrium), use Dashamula Taila, Ashwagandha Taila, almond oil or sesame oil as massage oils. For stimulating the pranic flow to the head and the body, apply aromatic oils like camphor, mint or eucalyptus, which open the mind and senses.
Treatment If Injured	Apply calamus powder with a little ghee for swelling. Wash the eyes (netra basti) with ghee for any accompanying inflammation or irritation of the eyes.

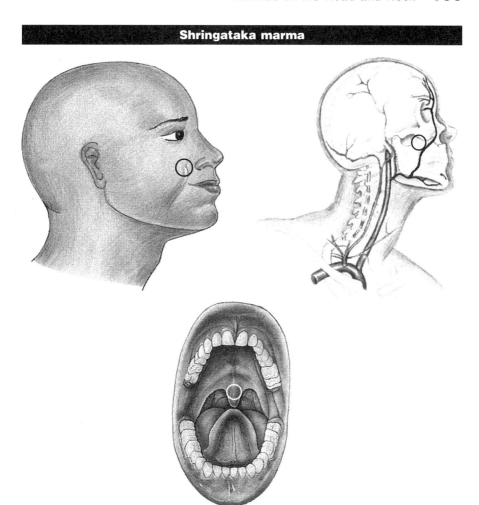

Shringataka marma

Shringataka

Description	
Name	Shringataka (place where four roads meet, a summit or horn)
Number	4 marma points
Type	Vessel (Sira)
Size	4 anguli (finger units)
Site	This is primarily an internal marma on the soft palate, which in yogic thought is the meeting point of the energies of the tongue, nose, eyes and ears. We can however work on the correspond-

	ing region of the face as per the illustration given above, the infraorbital foramen. It is another large marma region.
Controls	Controls Prana Vayu (primary vitality), Ojas (Soma), Tarpaka Kapha, Bodhaka Kapha (lubrication of the tongue) and the sense organ of taste, but also the senses of hearing, sight and smell. Here the subtle form of Kapha or Ojas provides nourishment to Prana and the mind.
Anatomical Structures	Supraorbital artery. Frontal diploic vein and superior sagital sinus. Occipito frontalis muscle. Ophthalmic nerve.
Qualities Relative to Injury	Sadya Pranahara (Immediate Death-Causing) type marma. Fiery in degree of vulnerability.
Symptoms If Injured	Injury will cause disorientation of the senses, hemorrhage and possible death.
Treatment	
Massage, Acupressure Aroma Therapy	Gently massage the corresponding area on the face. For Vata disorders, massage with Dashamula Taila, almond oil or sesame oil. Use nervine aromatic oils like calamus, myrrh, frankincense or mint to open up the powers of the senses. This marma is a good place for acupressure for treating diseases of the mouth. Use Kapha-reducing aromatic oils for this purpose like peppermint, cloves or calamus. We can also stimulate this point by sucking on spicy herbs like cloves or nutmeg, holding the herbs towards the back of the mouth.
Yoga and Meditation	The soft palate is an important place for concentration and meditation, said to give control over all the five senses and aid in the flow of Soma or nectar from the head (Sahasrara) chakra. It is called the place of the Moon (Soma or Kapha) opposite the place of the Sun (Agni or Pitta) in the navel. Meditation on this point improves contentment and peace of mind. The mantra SHRIM is good to use here for its nurturing, lunar energy.
Treatment If Injured	Combine turmeric powder with a little ghee and apply this paste at the injured area to relieve the pain and edema. Wash the eyes (netra basti) with ghee for any accompanying inflammation or irritation of the eyes.

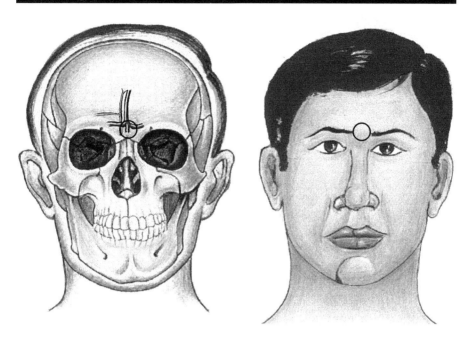

Sthapani marma

Sthapani

Description	
Name	Sthapani (what gives support or holds firm)
Number	1 marma point
Type	Vessel (Sira)
Size	1/2 anguli (finger unit)
Site	In between the eyebrows, the position of third eye (junction of the glabella of the frontal bone and the two nasal bones).
Controls	Controls the sixth chakra (Ajna), Prana, the mind, the senses, the pituitary gland, and the meeting of the six head nadis (Ida and Pingala, Pusha and Gandhari, Payasvini and Shankhini) in the Sushumna nadi. *Note:* The point in the middle of the forehead has similar properties but is stronger for controlling the mind, while Sthapani is better for controlling the senses. It governs the Agni of the mind and senses.

Anatomical Structures	Supraorbital and facial arteries, anterior facial vein, superior sagital sinus. Drainage to submandibular lymph glands. Supraorbital nerve. Frontal bone.
Qualities Relative to Injury	Vishalyaghna (Fatal If Pierced) type marma. Airy in degree of vulnerability.
Symptoms If Injured	Injury can easily damage Prana in the body as a whole as well as disturb the mind and senses.

Treatment

Massage, Acupressure and Aroma Therapy	Apply marma massage to the area, using a strong circular motion for about five minutes. This can be combined with general massage of the forehead. A good point for acupressure to calm and focus the mind. For treating disorders of the sixth chakra (Ajna) and Prana Vayu, massage with Dhanvantara Taila, Ashwagandha Taila, almond oil or plain sesame oil. This is a good site to apply shirodhara (oil drip to the head) using medicated sesame oils like Ashwagandha Taila or plain sesame oil. Sandalwood oil or paste applied here promotes meditation, calms the mind and nerves and relieves fever. Lotus aromatic oil is also good. Stimulating oils like camphor, bayberry, basil, mint or calamus open the mind and senses. Such aromatic oils work well, particularly if applied along with acupressure, which done at this point can release stress for the entire body and mind.
Yoga and Meditation	This is a key point in meditation for developing concentration, insight and focus for the mind and for unfolding the higher perceptual powers of the third eye. One can use the mantra OM for general energization purposes or the mantra AIM (pronounced 'I'm') for increasing powers of concentration. The yogic practice of trataka or fixing of the gaze energizes this marma, particularly, if one focuses on a ghee flame.
Treatment If Injured	If there is bleeding, apply ice and administer nasya (nasal application) of brahmi (gotu kola) juice or aloe gel. Take hemostatic herbs internally like brahmi (gotu kola) or turmeric, which work on the head. For pain, give pain-relieving herbs like calamus, brahmi or myrrh.

Simanta marma

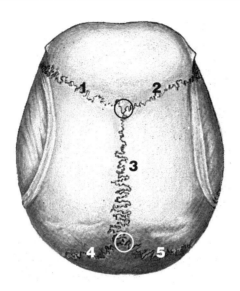

Simanta

Description	
Name	Simanta (the summit; the skull and surrounding joints)
Number	5 marma regions on the skull
Type	Joint (Sandhi)
Size	4 anguli (finger units)
Site	This marma consists of the sutures on the skull, so it is composed more of lines than points or regions and covers a large area. Its five components are the five aspects of these three sutures: the two sides of the coronal suture, the one sagital suture, and the two sides of the lambdoid suture.
Controls	Controls the seventh or head chakra (Sahasrara), nervous system, plasma, blood and circulatory systems (Majjavaha, Rasavaha and Raktavaha Srotamsi) as well as the mind and Prana, much like Adhipati marma, which marks its central point.
Anatomical Structures	Parietal-frontal, parietal-temporal and parietal-occipital joints. Occipito-frontalis muscle and epicranial apponeurosis. Opthalmic and maxillary nerves and second and third cervical

	nerves. Anterior and posterior superficial temporal and occipital arteries. Occipital diploic vein, posterior parietal, anterior parietal and frontal parietal veins.
Qualities Relative to Injury	Kalantara Pranahara (Long-term Death-Causing) type marma, owing to the protection afforded by the skull to the brain. Both fiery and watery in degree of vulnerability.
Symptoms If Injured	Injury may cause paralysis, hemorrhage or sudden death.

Treatment

Massage, Acupressure and Aroma Therapy	Massage with the fingers and the palm of the hands. A good method is to use the middle finger to go over all three sutures on the head. The two best points for acupressure in the Simanta area are where the sagital suture intersects the coronal suture in the front of the head and where it intersects the lambdoidal suture at the back of the head. Apply medicated oils like Dhanvantara Taila, Bhringaraj Taila, Ashwagandha Taila, almond oil or sesame oil for calming and relaxing purposes. Place gauze dipped in warm medicated oils like Dhanvantara Taila or sesame oil on the spot. To open the head energy, use etheric aromatic oils like camphor, mint or calamus. This is aided by the use of acupressure. For newborn children, warm sesame oil should be applied daily to this marma for controlling Vata, calming the nerves, promoting sleep and maintaining health.
Yoga and Meditation	Like Adhipati, chanting the mantra OM and meditating upon the head chakra improves all the functions of the top of the head region. Another method is to meditate upon the infinite expanse of space or the void extending from the top of the skull.
Treatment If Injured	For relieving pain and gaining consciousness, administer a virechana nasya (cleansing nasal application) of medicated calamus oil, or a snuff of calamus powder. Use consciousness-reviving aromatic oils like camphor, eucalyptus or ginger.

Adhipati marma

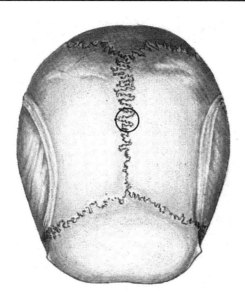

Adhipati

Description	
Name	Adhipati (the lord of all)
Number	1 marma point
Type	Joint (Sandhi)
Size	1/2 anguli (finger unit)
Site	Located on the vertex, the top point of the skull, on the sagital suture, just behind the anterior fontanelle, immediately superior to the external occipital protuberance. It is also the central point at the top of Simanta marma, so it has a ruling action over that marma as well and shares many of its properties. It is the soft spot on a baby's head.
Controls	Controls the seventh or head chakra (Sahasrara), pineal gland, nervous system (Majjavaha Srotas), Prana Vayu (primary vitality), Tarpaka Kapha (lubrication of the brain) and Sadhaka Pitta (thinking power), as well as Prana, Tejas and Ojas (primary factors of positive health, energy and vitality). It is the governing point of the entire body through the mind and brain, ruling over Prana as a whole. It relates to the transcendent or spiritual form of Agni.

Anatomical Structures	Occipito-parietal joint, occipital and parietal bones. Occipital artery, posterior diploic vein and occipital sagital sinus. Medulla oblongata and second and third cervical nerves.
Qualities Relative to Injury	Sadya Pranahara (Immediate Death-Causing) type marma. Fiery in degree of vulnerability.
Symptoms If Injured	Loss of consciousness, coma, injury to brain.

Treatment

Massage, Acupressure and Aroma Therapy	Apply marma massage to the area, using a strong circular motion, for about five minutes. It is also a good point for acupressure for calming and controlling the mind and emotions and opening higher perceptive powers. Use the index or middle finger for this purpose. The pressure can be strong. Sesame oil applied here calms Vata. Medicated oils like Ashwagandha Taila or Mahanarayan Taila are even better. The special Ayurvedic practice of Pichu dharana is good here. This consists of applying a gauze or piece of cotton dipped in medicated oils like Dhanvantara Taila or plain sesame oil. For treating Sadhaka Pitta (perceptive power of the brain), use Brahmi Taila and cooling aromatic oils like sandalwood, lotus, khus (vetiver) and chamomile. For treating Prana Vayu, use Dhanvantara Taila or sesame oil, or aromatic oils like basil, camphor and calamus. For treating Tarpaka Kapha, use sweet aromatic oils like jasmine, rose, lotus or gardenia. For stimulating the crown chakra use ether-containing aromatic oils like camphor or basil. In newborn children, the anterior fontanelle is open. Due to incomplete ossification, the top portion of the skull is only covered by a thin skin. For quick healing apply sesame oil daily to the site. This also nourishes Prana Vayu (primary vital energy) and calms the child.
Yoga and Meditation	Chanting the mantra OM and meditating upon the top of the head both energizes the higher mind and also helps us transcend the mind into the infinite space of pure consciousness. Meditation here also promotes deep and dreamless sleep and improves overall concentration, detachment and self-control.

Treatment If Injured	If the patient loses consciousness, have them snuff calamus or ginger powders in order to regain awareness or give them Hemagarbha Taila with ginger.
	Use awareness-promoting herbs and penetrating aromatic oils like asafoetida, camphor and eucalyptus, or the special Ayurvedic compound Brihat Vata Chintamani.

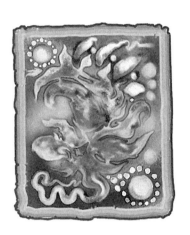

Part Three

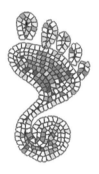

Supplemental Material and Appendices

Use of Instruments to Treat Marmas

The following materials deal with the third group of therapies introduced in Chapter 5, The Many Methods of Marma Therapy 1, which use various instruments to treat marma points. As these are mainly clinical procedures and as the explanation of them is only by way of outline, this material has been placed in the appendix. It is not meant to substitute for a full exposition of these important therapies.

While we will introduce acupuncture in this section, note that Appendix 2 contains a more detailed account of Marma-acupuncture also called 'Marmapuncture', puncturing of marma points by Frank Ros, an expert in that field.

1. Marma Therapy by Blood-letting

Ancient Ayurveda refers to the practice of 'vessel-piercing' (Sira Vedha), puncturing the different types of vessels through which Vata, Pitta, Kapha and blood flow. The most important type of this is piercing the blood vessels or blood-letting, called Rakta-moksha. Blood-letting is another important therapy in many systems of traditional medicine and in Ayurveda.[1] The piercing of small channels is more part of acupuncture as discussed in point number 2.

Blood-letting at specific locations and veins is an important part of Ayurvedic surgery and of marma therapy. It is counted among the methods of Pancha Karma (radical detoxification therapy). As a strong therapy, it should only be performed by therapists who are well-trained and on patients who possess suitable strength not to be weakened by the treatment (those whose Ojas is sufficient).

Blood-letting can involve cutting the skin (Pracchana or making abrasions with a small knife or needle) or taking blood from the veins (Sira Vedha or puncturing the veins with number 16 or 18 needles).[2] Another method not using instruments is with the help of leeches. This method is employed for infections such as boils and carbuncles.

Blood-letting is carried out on the visible veins. It is never done on the arteries. It should be done at the sensitive point nearest to the marma, which can be found by palpation. Blood-letting is indicated when Pitta and its subtypes are in excess, when the level of toxicity in the blood is high or for certain conditions of infection, inflammation or stagnant blood. Donating blood is often recommended for Pitta individuals because this type of therapy is helpful in a general way to keep Pitta in balance.

An alternative method to blood-letting, but milder in nature, is to apply blood-moving and alterative (blood-cleansing) herbs to marmas as well as to take them internally in the form of herbal teas and decoctions. Such blood-cleansing herbs include turmeric, myrrh, guggul, aloe, saffron, comfrey leaf, plantain, red clover, yellow dock and manjishta (madder).

2. Marma Therapy by Acupuncture (Suchi-karma)

Acupuncture, or using sharp instruments to treat marma points, has its counterpart in Ayurveda. There are ancient references to Suchi Veda, with Suchi meaning 'needle' and Veda meaning 'science'. As the piercing of marmas by weapons was found to cause great injury, it was thought that stimulating them using smaller pointed-instruments could improve the flow of Prana. In Ayurveda, acupuncture is commonly called Suchi-karma, or needle-therapy.

Acupuncture is part of Vyadhana or Bhedana Karma, referring to actions of 'cutting' or 'piercing' of marmas, blood-letting, and the puncturing of the smaller vessels that carry Prana and the doshas.[3] Sushruta mentions smaller channels (Keshavahinya or as thin as a hair), fine capillaries or minute vessels spread all over the body that carry the doshas. Acupuncture is done only on areas that contain small capillaries, where there can be no oozing of blood, but only a pacifying effect on the doshas.

For balancing the doshas, Sushruta advised puncturing the channels (sira), by using instruments as small as half a grain of rice.[4] These are needle numbers 26, 27 & 28 in size. With this needle the most sensitive point nearest to the center of the marma should be punctured.

Acupuncture on marmas should be avoided in conditions of skin diseases in the area of the procedure, during pregnancy and immediately after delivery. It should generally not be done on Sadya Pranahara (Immediate Death-Causing) marmas.

During the ancient period, bamboo or wooden needles were used for stimulating marma points. Later on, metal needles were developed for this purpose. Overall, however, the use of needles on marma points has been much less used in Ayurveda than in Chinese medicine and does not have a comparable sophistication.

Ayurvedic acupuncture is related to blood-letting and heat application (Agni-karma) methods and often used along with them. For those wishing to practice acupuncture on marma points, they should examine further information on the subject in Ayurvedic books.[5]

3. Marma Therapy by Agni-karma or Heat Therapy

Heat has powerful therapeutic properties, promoting circulation, improving digestion and stimulating healing. Heat therapy is called Agni-karma (fire-therapy) in Ayurveda. It involves heating and burning of the skin. For the application of heat, Sushruta advises various types of Shalakas or thin metal rods made from gold, silver, copper, iron or various alloys. This therapy is not applied to all marmas owing to its strong nature.[6]

Since marmas are sensitive areas, direct heat should not be used. Instead, one end of the metal rod should be applied to the sensitive point near the marma to be treated and the other end of the rod should be heated with a candle. The heat will travel from one end of the rod to the other. That amount of heat will be sufficient for treatment purposes. When treating marmas, one should apply high heat only to the level of the skin, not to that of the deeper muscle tissue.

Types of Agni-karma are classified according to the shape of the burn created by the type of rod used-pointed, half circle or circular. The point type is most commonly used in marma therapy. The marma is heated until it is slightly burned at a point.

Hot spicy herbs like ginger, cinnamon, cayenne, pippali, black pepper and mustard can be used for an 'herbal' Agni-karma. Pastes of these herbs can be placed on the marma for this purpose. Another method is a fomentation of the marma with a warm cloth soaked with the juices or aromatic oils of such hot-natured herbs. Aromatic oils from hot-natured herbs can also be applied to the site for the same effects. In this way, aroma therapy can be a method of heat application. For larger areas on the arms, legs or abdomen, heat lamps are good. Moxibustion is another method. Ayurveda uses herbs like calamus or turmeric, burning them on the marma (but taking care not to burn the skin).

Agni-karma (heat application) is particularly effective for arthritis, which often is caused by an accumulation of cold and dampness in the body, and for reducing Ama. For all types of joint pain, one should select the tenderest point closest to the marma.

Cold Application

The application of cold is not as important a therapeutic method as the application of heat because heat is better for stimulating and for cleansing marmas. However, it is still useful in many conditions.

Application of ice or cold packs is good for marmas where there is inflammation or bleeding. Fomentation using cooling herbs like sandalwood, cilantro (coriander leaves), comfrey leaves or licorice is very helpful in the same conditions. Cooling substances from cool water to cooling herbs like brahmi (gotu kola) are commonly applied to the top of the head, which benefits by being kept cool, particularly when there is fever. That is why the application of sandalwood oil to the forehead is so good for mental functioning and meditation. Aloe gel, another cooling herb, is similarly good to apply to marmas where there is burning or inflammation.

4. Marma Therapy by Kshara-karma (Application of Alkalis)

Ayurveda employs special medicated alkalis to treat marmas. These alkalis, called 'ksharas', have a chemically caused burning affect on the skin that stimulates the marma. This therapy is called Kshara-karma, or the alkali action,[7] much like the use of chemical cauterization in western medicine. It is regarded as another type of Agni-karma, or heat therapy. It is also a strong therapy that should only be done by those with the proper clinical training.

Ksharas are prepared from herbs dominant in the fire element, which affords them a penetrating action. Ksharas are white in color and act on all three doshas. They have a cleansing, stimulating and detoxifying effect. A medium strength Kshara is recommended for marma therapy. It should not be too strong so as to cause damage or too weak so as to have no effect.

---

[1] Note *Sushruta Samhita Sharira Sthana VIII* and *Sutra Sthana XIV.23-45* for a discussion of this topic.

[2] *Sushruta Samhita Sutrasthana XIV.25*

[3] Note *Sushruta Samhita Sharira Sthana VIII,* for an entire chapter on this topic.

[4] *Sushruta Samhita Sharira Sthana VIII.9.*

[5] Note *Ayurvedic Acupuncture* (Ros).

[6] Note *Sushruta Samhita Sutrasthana XII*, which chapter deals with this topic.

[7] Note *Sushruta Samhita Sutrasthana XI,* which chapter deals with this subject.

Marmapuncture, Ayurvedic Acupuncture

By Dr. Frank Ros

Recently, Ayurvedic researchers in India (Prof. Dr. Binod K. Joshi et al) have discovered that ancient Ayurvedic texts, specifically the *Sushruta Samhita,* contain much more information about marmas and acupuncture than was first perceived and included in the translations. Many of the terms used in the translations did not include the total subtlety or meaning of the words being translated.

As a consequence, these experts state: "Earlier interpretations of the *Sushruta Samhita* made mention of marmas, dhamanis and siras, which were believed to symbolize masses of tissue, arteries and veins, respectively. However, errors were made in the translation of those terms. In reviewing the treatise, evidence was found showing that the marmas correspond precisely with traditional acupuncture points used to treat the vital organs and that the dhamanis and siras depict meridians and channels that aid in the flow of qi. It was [previously] thought that the dhamanis and siras represent arteries and veins and, therefore, whenever damage used to occur, the first move was to preserve the concerned tissue. But then, these are actually the channels and meridians controlling the vital energy flow. Our conclusion is that the Sushruta Samhita is the base of acupuncture."[1]

In late 2001, experts in Sri Lanka headed by Prof. Dr. A. Jayasuriya, et al[2] discovered not only a long history of native acupuncture practice in Sri Lanka (something which is well known in Sri Lanka) but also the connotation that by archaeological evidence this area (including nearby India, the Kerala region) may have originated the practice of acupuncture. Only now are we discovering archaeological evidence of the early practice of acupuncture both in India and Sri Lanka possibly stemming from the Indus Valley civilization and certainly from Vedic times. A number of ancient acupuncture needles made of iron, copper and bronze were previously unearthed at the site of Taxila University, according to Prof. Dr. C.L. Nagpal.[3]

Even some ancient Indian Buddhist texts record acupuncture practice in India, including the *Chikitsa Vidya*.[4] Jivaka (Giba), the renowned Ayurvedic surgeon, was also considered a master acupuncturist in these texts. He was reputed "to have been born with an acupuncture needle in the right hand and a drug container in the left hand"[5], according to the *Chikitsa Vidya*.

Ayurvedic acupuncture is best called Marmapuncture because it aims at the puncturing of marma points. Like a number of other effective ancient Ayurvedic therapies, it fell into disuse much like the decline of Buddhism in India, its birthplace, and yet had meteoric development in the rest of the Orient. As in China prior to the onset of the Cultural Revolution, only a handful of families maintained the knowledge and practice of Marmapuncture in India.[6] Considering the cost involved in obtaining and maintaining expensive gold and silver needles (as no stainless steel was available), no wonder it fell into disrepair. It is only now with the advent of inexpensive stainless steel disposable needles that the practice of marmapuncture can develop into a popular art once again.

Marmapuncture is finely attuned to the same subtle concepts of diagnosis and treatment found in the other Ayurvedic modalities explained in this book. The fact that a traditional marmapuncturist will often utilize marma massage, heat therapy (Agni-karma) and Prana therapy (Prana Chikitsa) in conjunction with Marmapuncture means that these are all synergistic therapies reflecting the core of the system, which is Ayurveda.

The Ayurvedic perception that marmas should not be punctured stems back to the concept of surgery and injury to marmas during battles and wars. Kshatriyas, or warriors, would be treated by surgeons after their marmas had been traumatized during the process of fighting. This led many to the belief that marmas should not be punctured at all, even with acupuncture, in order to prevent the uninitiated from using the system and possibly causing injury. The concept of marmas was considered sacred and so this was also a means of keeping the knowledge secret. The definition of puncturing in this instance was the insertion of a sharp object in a forced or brutal way; for instance, a spear, knife or arrow that will cause major trauma or even death.

Marmapuncture, on the other hand, gives rise to controlled, minute trauma. Instead of inhibiting or killing the organism such as occurs in the case of a major, lethal trauma, this minor puncturing produces a stimulation that gently encourages the body into action for self-repair. This is not unlike the therapeutic use of aconite or arsenic in homeopathic doses compared to the lethal doses of the poison which would kill a person. It is aligned with law which states that the amount of dose (or trauma) relates to whether it kills (major dose), inhibits (medium dose) or stimulates (minute dose) the organism. This law is now also called hormesis in toxicology.

Sthapani and Hridaya marmas have been routinely needled by numerous practitioners since recorded history and yet no serious complications have occurred. However, these two marmas are regarded as lethal marmas because major trauma (brute puncturing) to them can cause serious problems.

However, certain marmas are not directly needled in marmapuncture. These include Nabhi (navel), Stanamula (nipples) and Nila (throat) marmas. Other marmas having similar qualities can be needled in their place or nearby points can be treated. Marmas located over sensitive organs and major arteries, which deep penetration may injure (like puncturing of the lung), are also generally avoided, especially by the inexperienced practitioner.

The major marmas that directly relate to the chakras should be needled very gently by rotating the needle as it is inserted. Guide tubes should not be used on these points because the tapping with the finger on the needle can affect both the marma and the chakra and aggravate the balance of the subtle body.

An expert marmapuncturist (suchika) utilizes the least number of needles to create the greatest therapeutic effect, with about fifteen needles being the maximum for one client. The number of needles also depends upon the client's body type as Vata, Pitta or Kapha.

Marmapuncture needles should normally be very fine (standard type is 0.25 mm x 25mm) as the thicker the needle the greater the potential to cause pain and aggravate Vata. Marmapuncture, therefore, is done with a careful attitude of not causing pain to the client and consequently does not involve the very deep insertion and strong manipulation of the needles. Needles are inserted into the marmas in a gentle and rhythmic way in accordance with the qualities of Vata, Pitta or Kapha and the body type of the client.

Because many marmas are classified as lethal sites, the area of the potential effect of the trauma is larger than the area of the insertion of the needle. For instance, Simanta marma on the summit of the head has an overall area of about four angulis, or finger units. Major trauma to any part of this area can cause a similar lethal effect (hemorrhage, paralysis or even death) irrespective of whether it occurs at the center or the periphery of the marma. In marmapuncture, the most appropriate place to needle in order to obtain the most subtle effect is usually at the center of the marma, although needling anywhere within the area of the marma will cause a similar effect (perhaps a more physical, related consequence). Because of this, many people regard marmas as larger than acupoints. Some experts avoid puncturing the center of the marma in order to avoid lethal effects but many years of practice also demonstrates that a therapeutic effect is best obtained when it is punctured correctly according to marmapuncture principles.

Modern research demonstrates that marmas are acupuncture points which have been needled for thousands of years without lethal effects. Lethal effects are caused by brute force puncturing of the marma, while needling of the periphery of the marma will create a therapeutic effect. Either way, whether needling at the periphery or the center of the marma, it is still effective. For instance, when treating subtle energies like the three gunas of Tamas, Rajas and Sattva or the vital essences of Prana, Tejas and Ojas, then the most subtle effect obtainable from the marma is generally desirable. When dealing with mainly physical diseases, then a more physical effect from a marma is desirable.

Marmapuncture Treatment

A marmapuncture treatment usually follows the appropriate Ayurvedic diagnosis where the conditions of the tissues, systems, Agni and Ojas are determined and an appropriate treatment plan is designed much the same way as for an Ayurvedic herbal therapy. A prescription of marma points is formulated to treat the factors out of balance.

There is a careful consideration of the three doshas (Vata, Pitta and Kapha) and appropriate points are included for these. There may also be a need to treat the mental aspect of the client (Sattva, Rajas and Tamas), so appropriate points for these may likewise be included. Treatment may include correctly adjusting the subdoshas in the appropriate direction, mainly Apana, Udana, Samana, Vyana and Prana Vayus but also Pitta and Kapha subdoshas. Consequently, most treatments cannot be textbook cases or mass-produced.

The final prescription or formula of marma points may contain a number of points that are duplicated because the same marma may have a multiple of qualities or effects. However, as a synergistic formula of points, the effect of the therapy is magnified because of the combination and not just because of the selection of individual points.

Needling Effects

The materials used for needling have their own qualities and effects on the doshas, so consequently attention should be paid where gold, silver or other materials are used. For instance, silver needles may aggravate Vata or Kapha on a subtle level. Gold may aggravate Pitta on a subtle level. Yet, the correct material for the person's body type will enhance the therapy, especially on a subtle level and to treat psychological or emotional imbalances.

Needles are kept inserted according to the client's body type, with Vata clients requiring less time than Pitta or Kapha. Kapha requires the most time. The usual marmapuncture treatment may take up to an hour, the length depending on the body type or constitution of the client.

The techniques used may aggravate or improve the client according to his/her body type. Strong, erratic actions will aggravate Vata but may improve a Kapha disorder. Smooth, slow actions may not assist a Kapha person as these will add to the qualities of Kapha and hence its aggravation.

Needling Effects According to Doshas

REQUIREMENT	DOSHA
Marma Depth of Insertion	
Shallow	Vata
Medium	Pitta
Deeper	Kapha
Number of Needles	
Minimum	Vata
Medium	Pitta
Most	Kapha
Needle Material	
Gold or Silver	Vata
Silver	Pitta
Gold	Kapha
Needling Action/Insertion	
Gentle, rhythmic	Vata
Medium rhythmic	Pitta
Erratic, strong	Kapha
Needling Time	
15-30 mins	Vata
20-40 mins	Pitta
40-60 mins	Kapha
Electric Pulse	
Slow, rhythmic, less intense	Vata
Medium, regular, rhythmic	Pitta
Intense, fast, erratic	Kapha
Agni-karma (Heat Application)	
May require heat but not excessive	Vata
Does not generally require heat	Pitta
May require heat	Kapha

Marmas and Marmapuncture

Marmas are energy wells and energy wheels connected by a meridian system of conduits (nadis) with organs and other parts of the body. They are generally more physical than the chakras, which are more energy centers of the subtle body. By needling marmas, the energy flow through these channels can be corrected and a balance brought to the human organism. This balance of energy equates with health. Marmas can be injured or they can be healed, depending on the amount of trauma caused, much the same way that gentle, controlled pressure from massage can help heal while massive pressure from a blow can cause injury. Marmas are:

- Vulnerable points on the body, susceptible to injury.
- Regarded as the physical and external aspect of the body's defense mechanism or immune system.
- Considered as a form of energy wheels and energy wells.
- A terminus for the pranic flow from the related organ through its nadi or related pranic channel.
- Sites for interchanging pranic energy from the outside (macrocosm) to the inside (microcosm) of the body through the skin.
- An area on the skin with lower galvanic skin resistance.
- Sites of Sattva, Rajas and Tamas; Vata, Pitta and Kapha; and the Five Elements.
- The external reflection of the chakras.
- Therapeutic points.

Besides the 107 major marmas considered by Ayurveda as lethal (or with potentially lethal effects) there are many other marmas that have been traditionally used both in marmapuncture and Indian martial arts (Kalaripayyat). At least 220 marmas are used in Kalaripayyat,[7] with at least 360 marmas used in one form or another in marmapuncture. Many of the not so lethal marmas are classified and named under their effects or their locations. For instance, there is an Apana marma located several finger units (angulis) above the malleolus, inside of the leg. This point or marma has a therapeutic effect on Apana Vayu energy. There is also an Udana marma located several finger units above the wrist crease on the inside of the arm. This marma balances Udana Vayu. The Five Elements themselves have marmas that directly relate and treat these elements. Some of these marmas are outside of the 107-marma system.

Accordingly, marmas have a number of therapeutic effects and can be used for various problems. In clinical practice, only about fifty to sixty marmas are regularly used, although this number will vary according to the problem and body type of the client. There are times when other marmas with specific qualities are required for treatment because of the seriousness or specific nature of the disease.

Since the 1970's some marmapuncture practitioners have used the modern international convention of numbering acupoints (e.g. Sthapani marma = G 24.5). This new system has been found useful in teaching by providing a clear, shortcut system, much like shorthand writing. However, the traditional names are still retained and used just like they are in Chinese acupuncture today.

Akashic Balancing

Treatment of the most subtle or etheric aspects (akasha) of the person in order to facilitate the free flow of Prana is the aim of Akashic Balancing. This is a technique using marmapuncture, pranic therapy (Prana chikitsa) and essential aromas/tastes to balance the psychological and emotional states or koshas of the body. Disease is considered a restriction of Prana or energy through the body, so the more restriction is encountered by Prana along its pathways (nadis), the more serious or deeper is the health problem. This is akin to the analogy of an electric radiator element that has a high resistance to the flow of electricity, causing friction, heat and light to generate. In a radiator this is the desired effect but in the human body it results in disease. Like a pure gold wire conductor (e.g. gold wire tracks on computer circuit boards), where the electricity has a free flow allowing the signals to arrive at their intended destination, Prana also requires an unimpeded path.

Akashic Balancing is helpful to produce clarity and focus in thoughts and ideas as well as for peak physical achievement. In Akashic Balancing all five Pranas are treated at the same time in order to stimulate the proper flow and direction of Prana. However, only after proper marmapuncture treatment for normal physical complaints is completed and any physical disease symptoms are removed should Akashic Balancing be attempted. Then the body is prepared for this special type of treatment, which is very different from the previous normal marmapuncture. Most clients of this method relate feeling totally different than the conventional acupuncture/marmapuncture treatment. There is generally a sense of lightness, positivity and mental clarity as well as an overall feeling of well-being.

---

[1] *The Hindu*, Dr. Binod K. Joshi, Dr. Ram L. Shah, et al., April 2001.

[2] *The Daily News*, Prof. Dr. A. Jayasuriya et al., Sri Lanka, July 27, 2001.

[3] *Modern Acupuncture*, Prof. Dr. C.L.Nagpal, A.S.I. Publications: Jaipur, India (pp. 3-4).

[4] *Acupuncture Medicine*, Yoshiaki Omura D.Sc. MD, Japan Publications Inc., Tokyo, Japan, 1982 (p.15)

[5] Ibid.

[6] *Tao and Dharma*, Dr. Robert Svoboda and Arnie Lade, Lotus Press, 1995 (p.144).

[7] *Ayurveda, Life, Health and Longevity*, Dr. Robert Svoboda, Arkana Penguin Books, London, 1992.

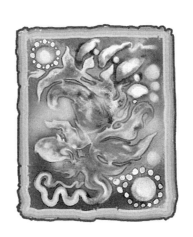

Names and Classifications of Marmas

Marmas and Their Sanskrit Names

Most of these are anatomical in nature but a few have specialized meanings reflecting their effects.

Adhipati—overlord; because it rules over the brain and head; crown of the head

Amsaphalaka—shoulder blade; reflecting its anatomical position

Amsa—shoulder; reflecting its anatomical position

Ani—the point of a needle; reflecting its powerful affect, the lower region of the upper arm or leg

Apalapa—unguarded; reflecting its vulnerability, the armpit or axilla

Apanga—the outer corner of the eyes; reflecting its anatomical position

Apastambha—standing to the side; a point on the upper abdomen said to carry Prana or the life-force

Avarta—calamity; from its sensitiveness; the point above the center of each eye

Bahvi—what relates to the arm; reflecting its anatomical position

Basti—bladder; reflecting its anatomical position, the lower abdomen

Brihati—the large or the broad region of the back; reflecting its anatomical form

Guda—anus; reflecting its anatomical position

Gulpha—ankle joint; reflecting its anatomical position

Hridaya—heart; reflecting its anatomical position

Indrabasti—Indra's arrow or a superior type of arrow; owing to the shape of the muscles in the region; a point on the lower arm or lower leg. Basti also means bladder in other contexts.

Janu—Knee joint; reflecting its anatomical location

Kakshadhara—what upholds the flank; reflecting its physiological effects, the top of the shoulder joint

Katikataruna—what rises from the hip; reflecting its anatomical position near the hip joint

Krikatika—joint of the neck; reflecting its anatomical location

Kshipra—quick; reflecting its immediate effect, points between the thumb and index finger on the hand and between the big toe and first toe on the foot

Kukundara—marking the loins; reflecting its location on either side of posterior superior iliac spines

Kurcha—a knot or bundle; reflecting the knot of muscles at the base of the thumb or big toe

Kurchashira—the head of kurcha; reflecting its connection to kurcha marma, which it is located below at the root of the thumb or big toe

Kurpara—elbow joint; reflecting its anatomical position

Lohitaksha—red-jointed as it is a point for the blood and the hip and shoulder joints; the lower frontal end of the shoulder joint and hip joint

Manibandha—bracelet; reflecting its connection to the wrist

Manya—honor; owing to its connection with the voice, a point on the upper side of the neck

Nabhi—navel or umbilicus; reflecting its anatomical position

Nila—dark blue; from the color of the nearby veins at the base of the neck

Nitamba—the buttocks; reflecting its anatomical position

Parshvasandhi—the side of the waist; reflecting its anatomical position

Phana—serpent's hood; reflecting its anatomical structure, the side of the nostrils

Shankha—conch; reflecting the temple

Shringataka—place where four roads meet; owing to the crossroads of the senses that exists at the soft palate of the mouth

Simanta-summit; reflecting its anatomical position on the skull

Sira Matrika-mother of the blood vessels; owing to its connection with the common carotid artery in the lower neck region

Stanamula—root of the breast; reflecting its anatomical position

Stanarohita—upper region of the breast; reflecting its anatomical position

Sthapani—what gives support or fixes; reflecting its connection with the power of concentration, the point between the eyes

Talahridaya—center of the sole or palm; reflecting its anatomical position

Utkshepa—what is cast upwards; owing to its location above the ears

Urvi—what is wide; reflecting its anatomical structure, the wide region of the thighs

Vidhura—distress; due to its sensitiveness, a point below and behind the ears

Vitapa—hot or painful; reflecting its sensitive nature, the perineum, where the legs are connected to the trunk

Categories of Marmas

A. According to Anatomical Factors		
1. Mamsa-*Muscle*	11 Marmas	4 Indrabasti, 4 Talahridaya, 2 Stanarohita, 1 Guda
2. Sira- *Vessel (Arteries and Veins)*	41 Marmas	2 Brihati, 8 Sira Matrika, 2 Nila, 2 Manya, 2 Phana, 1 Hridaya, 1 Nabhi, 2 Parshvasandhi, 2 Stanamula, 2 Apalapa, 1 Sthapani, 2 Urvi, 2 Bahvi, 2 Apastambha, 4 Lohitaksha, 2 Apanga, 4 Shringataka
3. Snayu - *Ligaments and Tendons*	27 Marmas	4 Ani, 4 Kurcha, 4 Kurchashira, 4 Kshipra, 2 Amsa, 2 Utkshepa, 1 Basti, 2 Vitapa, 2 Kakshadhara, 2 Vidhura
4. Asthi-*Bone*	8 Marmas	2 Katikataruna, 2 Nitamba, 2 Amsaphalaka, 2 Shankha
5. Sandhi-*Joint*	20 Marmas	2 Janu, 2 Kurpara, 5 Simanta, 1 Adhipati, 2 Gulpha, 2 Manibandha, 2 Kukundara, 2 Avarta, 2 Krikatika
6. Dhamani-*Nerve*	9 Marmas	1 Guda, 2 Apastambha, 2 Vidhura, 4 Shringataka (This is a special classification, not found in Sushruta but only in Vagbhatta (Ashtanga Hridaya). Sushruta places these marmas in the other categories)

B. According to Region of the Body

1. Arms and hands	11 Marma Regions 22 Marma Points	2 Kshipra, 2 Talahridaya, 2 Kurcha, 2 Kurchashira, 2 Manibandha, 2 Indrabasti, 2 Kurpara, 2 Ani, 2 Bahvi, 2 Lohitaksha, 2 Kakshadhara
2. Legs and feet	11 Marma Regions 22 Marma Points	2 Kshipra, 2 Talahridaya, 2 Kurcha, 2 Kurchashira, 2 Gulpha, 2 Indrabasti, 2 Janu, 2 Ani, 2 Urvi, 2 Lohitaksha, 2 Vitapa
3. Abdomen and Chest	8 Marma Regions 12 Marma Points	1 Guda, 1 Basti, 1 Nabhi, 1 Hridaya, 2 Stanamula, 2 Stanarohita, 2 Apalapa, 2 Apastambha
4. On the Back and Hips	7 Marma Regions 14 Marma Points	2 Katikataruna, 2 Kukundara, 2 Nitamba, 2 Parshvasandhi, 2 Brihati, 2 Amsa, 2 Amsaphalaka
5. On the Neck and Head	14 Marma Regions 37 Marma Points	2 Krikatika, 2 Vidhura, 2 Phana, 2 Apanga, 2 Avarta, 2 Utkshepa, 2 Shankha, 2 Nila, 2 Manya, 1 Sthapani, 1 Adhipati, 5 Simanta, 4 Shringataka, 8 Sira Matrika

C. According to Size

1. One finger breadth *(1 anguli)*	Total 12	2 Urvi, 2 Bahvi, 4 Kurchashira, 2 Vitapa, 2 Kakshadhara
2. Two finger breadths *(2 anguli)*	Total 6	2 Gulpha (ankle), 2 Manibandha, 2 Stanamula
3. Three finger breadths *(3 anguli)*	Total 4	2 Janu (knee), 2 Kurpara (elbow)
4. Fist size or Four finger breadth *(4 anguli)*	Total 29	4 Kurcha, 1 Guda (anus), 1 Basti (bladder), 1 Nabhi (navel), 1 Hridaya (heart), 2 Nila, 2 Manya, 8 Sira Matrika, 5 Simanta, 4 Shringataka
5. One half finger breadth *(1/2 anguli)*	Total 56	4 Kshipra, 4 Talahridaya, 4 Indrabasti, 4 Ani, 4 Lohitaksha, 2 Apalapa, 2 Apastambha, 2 Katikataruna, 2 Kukundara, 2 Nitamba, 2 Parshvasandhi, 2 Brihati, 2 Amsa, 2 Amsaphalaka, 2 Stanarohita, 2 Krikatika, 2 Vidhura, 2 Phana, 2 Apanga, 2 Avarta, 2 Utkshepa, 2 Shankha, 1 Sthapani, 1 Adhipati

D. According to Symptoms If Injured		
Type	**Number**	**Specific Marmas**
1. Sadya Pranahara *(Immediate Death-Causing or fiery)*	19	4 Shringataka, 1 Adhipati, 2 Shankha (temples), 8 Sira-Matrika, 1 Guda (anus), 1 Hridaya (heart), 1 Basti (bladder), 1 Nabhi (navel)
2. Kalantara Pranahara *(Long-term Death-Causing or both fiery and watery)*	33	4 Talahridaya, 4 Kshipra, 4 Indrabasti, 2 Apalapa, 2 Apastambha, 2 Stanarohita, 2 Stanamula, 5 Simanta, 2 Katikataruna, 2 Parshvasandhi, 2 Brihati, 2 Nitamba
3. Vishalyaghna *(Fatal If Pierced or airy)*	3	2 Utkshepa, 1 Sthapani
4. Vaikalyakara *(Disability-Causing or watery)*	44	4 Lohitaksha, 4 Ani, 2 Janu (knee), 2 Urvi, 2 Bahvi, 4 Kurcha, 2 Vitapa, 2 Kurpara, 2 Kukundara, 2 Kakshadhara, 2 Vidhura, 2 Krikatika, 2 Amsa (shoulder), 2 Amsaphalaka, 2 Apanga, 2 Nila, 2 Manya, 2 Phana (nostrils), 2 Avarta
5. Rujakara *(Pain-causing or both fiery and airy)*	8	2 Manibandha, 4 Kurchashira, 2 Gulpha (ankle)

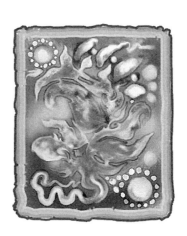

Sanskrit
Ayurvedic Terms

Abhyanga—Massage

Agni—specifically, the digestive fire; generally, fire as a cosmic principle

Agni-karma—Heat therapy

Alochaka—Pitta in the eyes

Ama—Toxins in the digestive tract, as opposed to the doshas, which are more specific toxins

Ambhuvaha Srotas—see Udakavaha Srotas

Annavaha Srotas—Channels carrying food, or the digestive system

Anguli—Finger unit

Apana Vayu—Downward-moving form of Vata

Asthi—Bone tissue

Asthivaha Srotas—Channels carrying bone or skeletal system

Atman—Higher Self

Avalambaka—Form of Kapha in the chest

Basti—Enema therapy; bathing an area with herbs or oils; also refers to the bladder

Bhrajaka Pitta—Pitta in the skin

Bodhaka Kapha—Form of Kapha on the tongue

Brimhana—Tonification or tissue-building therapy

Chakra—Energy center of the subtle body

Charaka—Important ancient Ayurvedic teacher

Chikitsa—Therapy

Dhamani—Vessel, generally nerve

Dhanur Veda—Vedic martial arts

Dhara—Pouring or dripping of oils onto a particular site, usually the forehead

Dhatu—Tissue

Dosha—Biological humor

Ghrita—Ghee (clarified butter)

Gunas—Prime qualities of nature as sattva, rajas and tamas

Ida nadi—Left nostril channel

Jatharagni—Digestive fire

Kapha—Biological water-humor

Kledaka Kapha—Form of Kapha in the stomach

Kshara-karma—The use of caustic herbal alkalis

Kundalini—Serpent power; energy source for the subtle body

Langhana—Reduction therapy

Lepa—Herbal paste

Majja—Nerve tissue

Majjavaha Srotas—Channels carrying nerve impulses or nervous system

Mala—Waste-material

Mamsa—Muscle tissue

Mamsavaha Srotas—Channels carrying the muscles or muscular system

Mani—Gem

Mani Chikitsa—Gem therapy

Manovaha Srotas—Channels carrying thought or the mind

Mantra—Sacred sounds for healing the mind and promoting meditation

Mantra Chikitsa—Mantra therapy

Mardana—Acupressure or pressure-based massage

Marma—Pressure point or sensitive region

Marma Vidya—Science of marma

Marma Chikitsa—Marma therapy

Meda—Fat tissue

Medovaha Srotas—Channels carrying fat or the adipose system

Mutravaha Srotas-Urinary system

Nadi—Subtle pranic channels of which 14 are most important

Nasya—Nasal application of herbs, oils or liquids

Ojas—Master form of Kapha as power of immunity and endurance

Pachaka Pitta—Form of Pitta in the digestive system

Pancha Karma—The five methods of Ayurvedic purification, or Shodhana therapy, as vamana or vomiting, virechana or purgatives, basti or enemas, nasya or nasal medications, and raktamoksha or blood-letting

Pingala nadi—Right nostril channel

Pitta—Biological fire-humor

Prakriti—Nature; matter or manifestation principle, constitution

Prana—Primary life-force

Prana Chikitsa—Prana therapy

Pranavaha Srotas—Channels carrying Prana, or the respiratory system

Pranayama—Extending the Prana, breath control exercises

Pratyahara—Yogic methods of sensory control and interiorization of the mind

Purusha—Consciousness principle, higher Self

Purishavaha Srotas—Excretory system

Rajas—Quality of Aggression

Rakta—Blood

Raktavaha Srotas—Channels carrying blood or circulatory system

Ranjaka—Form of Pitta in the liver and blood

Rasa—Plasma and lymphatics

Rasavaha Srotas—Channels carrying the plasma or lymphatic system

Rasayana—Rejuvenation therapy

Sadhaka Pitta—Form of Pitta in the brain

Samana Vayu—Balancing air

Sattva—Quality of balancing, harmonizing or healing

Shamana—Palliation or calming therapy, particularly for improving digestion and removing toxins from the digestive tract (Ama)

Shodhana—Cleansing or detoxification therapy, particularly of the doshas

Shukra—Reproductive tissues

Shukravaha Srotas—Reproductive system

Siddha Tradition—South Indian yogic and healing tradition connected to Ayurveda

Sira—Vessel, generally blood-vessel

Sira Vedha or Sira Vyadhana—Blood-letting, literally 'vessel-piercing'

Sleshaka Kapha—Form of Kapha in the joints

Snayu—Ligament

Snehana—Ayurvedic oil therapy, including oil massage

Srotas—Channel system of the body

Srotamsi—plural of srotas

Suchi—karma-Acupuncture

Sushruta—Important ancient Ayurvedic teacher

Sweda—Sweat

Swedana—Ayurvedic sweating therapy

Swedavaha Srotas—Sweating system, sebaceous glands

Taila—Ayurvedic medicated oil, generally sesame oil based, with various herbs cooked in the oil

Tamas—Quality of inertia

Tantra—Yogic tradition of energy practices using body and mind

Tarpaka Kapha—Form of Kapha in the brain and nervous system

Tejas—Master form of Pitta as positive force of fire and vitality

Udakavaha Srotas—Water-metabolism system, water intake portion of digestive system

Udana Vayu—Upward-moving air

Vagbhatta—Important ancient Ayurvedic teacher

Vajikarana—Promoting vitality and sexual energy

Varma—Same as marma but as a place that requires protection

Vata—Biological air-humor

Vayu—Form of Prana or Vata; particularly the five Vayus of Prana, Apana, Udana, Samana and Vyana

Vedic science—Spiritual and sacred sciences through the Vedic and Yoga traditions

Virechana—Detoxification or purgation therapy

Virechana Nasya—cleansing nasal application

Vyana Vayu-Outward—moving air

Yoga—Vedic science of physical and mental discipline aiming at Self-realization

Yoga Chikitsa—Yoga therapy

Herbs and Oils

A. Special Ayurvedic Herbs and Botanical Names

(Note that we have not listed the botanicals for the common western herbs listed in the text, for this consult any good western herbal text, also note *The Yoga of Herbs* by Frawley and Lad)

Agaru—Aquilaria agalocha

Agnimantha—Premna integrefolia

Amalaki—Emblica officinalis

Amruta—see Guduchi

Apamarga—Achryanthus aspera

Arjuna—Terminalia arjuna

Arka—Calotropis gigantean

Ashoka—Saraca indica

Ashwagandha—Withania somnifera

Atibala—Sida rhombifolia

Bala—Sida cordifolia

Bhallatak—Semicarpus anacardium

Bhringaraj—Eclipta alba

Bhunimba—Swertia chirata

Bibhitaka—Terminalia belerica

Bilva—Aegle marmelos, bael

Brahmi—Centella asiatica, gotu kola

Brihati—Solanum indicum

Cedarwood—Juniperus virginiana, juniper

Chandana—Santalum album, sandalwood

Chitraka—Plumbago zeylonica

Davana—Artemesia pallens

Deodar/ Devadaru—Cedrus deodar, Himalayan cedar

Durva—Cyndon dactylon

Ela—Eletteria cardamomum, cardamom

Elemi—Canarium luzonicum

Eranda—Ricinus communis, castor bean

Galbanum (ferula species).

Geranium—Pelargonium ordorantissium

Gojihva—Onosmum bractatum

Gokshura—Tribulus terrestris

Guduchi—Tinospora cordifolia

Guggul—Commiphora mukul

Haritaki—Terminalia chebula

Heena—Lawsonia inermis, aromatic oil of henna

Himalayan cedarwood—Cedrus deodar

Jatamamsi —Nardostachys jatamamsi

Jeeraka—Cumin, Carum carvi

Jivanti—Leptadenia reticulata

Jyotishmati—Celastrus paniculata

Kadamba—Anthocephalus kadamba

Kankola—Piper cubeba, cubebs

Kantakari—Solanum xanthocarpum

Kapikacchu—Mucuna pruriens

Karpasa—Gossypium herbaceum, cotton

Karpura—Camphor

Karaja—Pongamia glabra

Katphala—Myrica nagi, bayberry

Khus—see Ushira

Kutki—Picorrhiza kurroa

Kumkuma—Crocus sativus, saffron

Kushtha—Saussurea lappa

Kushmanda—Benincasa hispida

Laksha—Lacifera lacca

Lashuna—Garlic

Lavanga—Syzgium aromaticum, cloves

Lodhra—Symplocus racemosus

Madhuka—Madhuka indica

Manjishtha—Rubia cordifolia, madder

Masha—Phaseolus roxburghii

Mogra—Murraya paniculata

Mocharas—Bombax malabaricus

Musli—Asparagus adescendens

Musta—Cyperus rotundus, nutgrass

Nagakeshara—Messua ferrea

Nimba—Azadirechta indica

Neem—see nimba

Nirgundi—Vitex negundo

Padmaka—Prunus cerasoides

Padma—Nelumbo nucifera, lotus

Parpata—Fumaria pervaiflora

Patola—Trichosanthes cucumeria

Pippali—Piper longum

Plaksha—Ficus lacor

Prasarini—Paederia foetida

Punarnava—Boerrhavia diffusa

Rasna—Pleuchea lanceolata

Sahachara—Barleria prionitis

Sahadevi—Vernonia cinerea

Sariva—Cryptolepis buchanani

Shala—Shorea robusta

Shallaki—Boswellia serrata

Shalmali—Salmalia malabarica

Shankhapushpi—Crotalaria verrucosa

Shatavari—Asperagus racemosus

Shigru—Moringa pterigosperma

Shilajit—Shilajita (a mineral)

Shunthi—Zingiber officinalis, ginger

Tagara—Valerian

Triphala—Three myrobalans, haritaki, bibhitaka and amalaki

Tulsi—Ocinum sanctum

Udumbara—Ficus religeosa

Ushira—Vetivera zizanoides or Andropogon muricatus, khus

Vacha—Acorus calamus, calamus

Vamsha rochana—Bambusa arundinaceae

Vasa—Adhatoda vasika

Vatsanabha—Aconitum ferox

Vetiver—Vetivera zizanoides, note Ushira

Vidanga—Embelia ribes

Vidari—Ipomea digitata

Yashtimadhu—Licorice

B. Ayurvedic Medicated Oils (Tailas) and Herbal Formulas

1. Agaru Taila—Agaru, bilva, licorice and sesame oil (BR)

2. Amla or Amalaki Taila—Amalaki, haritaki, bibhitaka, bilva, sariva, ela and sesame oil (BR)

3. Amrita Taila—Tinispora cordifolia, triphala and sesame oil (BR)

4. Anu Taila—Licorice, other herbs and sesame oil

5. Arjuna Taila—Decoction of the bark of arjuna and sesame oil (BR)

6. Asana-eladi Taila—Asana, ela, jivanti, bilva, bala roots, deodara, sesame oil (SY)

7. Asana-bilvadi Taila—Asana, bilva, bala, amruta, camphor, milk, coconut oil (SY)

8. Ashwagandhadi Taila—Ashwagandha and sesame oil

9. Bala Taila—Bala, guduchi, rasna, ela, agaru, manjishtha, atibala, licorice, tulsi, cloves, kankola, nagakeshara and sesame oil (AH)

10. Bilvadi Taila—Bilva and sesame oil (BR)

11. Brahmi Taila—Brahmi and coconut oil (BR)

12. Brihat Marma Gutika—Pill composed of extracts of vidari, jivanti, shatavari, musta, amalaki, sariva, guduchi and durva, triturated with a decoction of gokshura and ushira. Then powders of licorice, red and white sandalwood are added to make the tablets. Dosage is 50 milligrams three times a day for 15 days (SY)

13. Brihat Saindhavadi Taila—Rock salt (saindhava), arka, black pepper, chitraka, turmeric and sesame oil (BR)

14. Bhringaraj oil—Eclipta alba, manjishtha, lodhra, bala, barberry, licorice, sandalwood, and sesame oil (BR)

15. Bhringamalakadi Taila—Juice of bhringaraj and amalaki, licorice, milk and sesame oil (SY)

16. Chandanadi Taila—Sandalwood, licorice, khus, jatamamsi, agaru, bala, bilva, kutki, sesame oil (YR)

17. Chandan-bala-lakshadi Taila—Red and white sandalwood, bala root, laksha, madhuka, devadaru, manjishtha, agaru, ashwagandha, rasna and sesame oil (YR)

18. Dashamula Taila—Dashamula (ten special roots) and sesame oil

19. Devadarvyadi Taila—Devadaru (Himalayan cedar) and sesame oil

20. Dhanvantara Kashaya—Decoction of bala root, dashamula, sariva, valerian, calamus, punarnava, manjishta, sandalwood, jaggery and honey.

21. Dhanvantara Taila—Bala roots, cow's milk, kushtha, bilva, patala, agaru, sandalwood, calamus, punarnava, licorice, sariva, haritaki, amalaki (AH and Vaidya Yogaratnavali)

22. Durvadi Taila—Durva, nimba, narikala ksheera, licorice and coconut oil (AH)

23. Gandha Taila—herbs in kakolyadi group (kakoli, kshira kakoli, black gram, medha, mahameda, guduchi, jivanti, kakadshingi, vamsha-rochana) cow's milk and sesame oil (AH)

24. Himasagara Taila—Shatavari, kushmanda, vidari, valerian, sandalwood, manjishtha, agaru, licorice, lodhra, musta, shalmali and sesame oil (BR)

25. Jirakadi Taila—Cumin and sesame oil

26. Jyotishmati Taila—Jyotishmati and apamarga (YR)

27. Karpas-asthyadi Taila—Cotton seeds, bala, masha, rasna, deodaru, punarnava, shigru, kushtha, coconut oil (SY)

28. Karpuradi Taila—Camphor and other herbs in sesame oil

29. Kshara Taila—Plant alkali of apamarga, calamus, ginger, kushtha, deodaru and sesame oil (BR)

30. Kshirabala Taila—Bala roots, cow's milk, sesame oil (AH)

31. Kottamachukadi Taila—Kushtha, musta, calamus, garlic, deodaru, sesame oil (SY)

32. Kumkumadi Taila—Saffron, ushira, laksha, sandalwood, licorice, nagakeshara, manjishtha, sesame oil

33. Laghu Marma Gutika—Pill prepared with extracts of shatavari, amalaki, guduchi, musli, both types of sandalwood and licorice. To this is added shilajit and the mixture is triturated with the decoction of bark of various plants and made into tablets. The dosage is 100 milligrams three times a day for 15 days.

34. Lakshadi Taila—Laksha, turmeric, manjishtha and sesame oil (BR)

35. Lashunadi Taila—garlic and sesame oil

36. Mahamanjishtadi Taila—Manjishtha, bilva, Agnimantha, patala, brihati, bala, rasna, ashwagandha, punarnava, atibala, sandalwood, manjishtha, kushtha, ela, musta, camphor, sesame oil (BR)

37. Mahamasha Taila—Masha, dashamula, calamus, black pepper, gokshura and sesame oil (BR)

38. Mahanarayan Taila—Bilva, ashwagandha, brihati, gokshura,, bala, kantakari, atibala, rasna, deodaru, agaru, haritaki, cardamom, licorice, calamus, sesame oil (BR)

39. Manjishtadi Taila—Manjishtha, sariva, musta, kutki, nutmeg, triphala, kushtha, jatamamsi, aloe juice and sesame oil (SY)

40. Marma Kashaya—Decoction containing ten roots: castor root, kushtha, licorice, ushira, nagakeshara, vasa, kapikacchu, guggul, rasna and ashwagandha.

41. Masha Taila—Masha and sesame oil

42. Nalapamaradi Taila—Juice of fresh curcuma, parpata, udumbara, plaksha, triphala, agaru, kushtha, and sesame oil (SY)

43. Narayan Taila—Shatavari, dashamula, punarnava, ashwagandha, kantakari, jatamamsi, calamus, kushtha, milk and sesame oil (BR)

44. Nimba Taila—Juice of leaves of nimba and sesame oil

45. Nimbapatradi Taila—Juice of leaves of nimba, bhringaraj, shatavari, manjishtha, licorice, ushira, musta, amruta, sariva, milk and sesame oil (SY)

46. Nirgundi Taila (Shefali oil)—Juice of nirgundi and sesame oil

47. Panchamla Taila—Sesame oil and five sour plants

48. Padmakadi Taila—Lotus stem, durva, sesame oil.

49. Pinda Taila—Bee's wax, manjishtha, sarjarasa, sariva, dhanyamla, sesame oil (AH)

50. Sahachara Taila—Sahachara, bilva, gokshura, sandalwood, shilajat, and sesame oil (AH)

51. Shankhapushpi Taila—Shankhapushpi, bilva, agaru and sesame oil

52. Shatadhauta Ghrita—specially prepared ghee in a copper vessel and washed with water

53. Shatavari Taila—Shatavari and sesame oil

54. Triphala Ghrita—Triphala and ghee

55. Triphaladi Taila—Triphala, guduchi, bala, castor, kushtha, ushira, musta, milk, sesame oil (SY)

56. Ushiradi Taila—Vetiver, other herbs and sesame oil

57. Vacha Taila—Calamus, haritaki, laksha, kutki and sesame oil

58. Vacha-lashunadi Taila—Calamus, garlic and sesame oil

59. Vishagarbha Taila—Datura alba, kushtha, vatsanabha, calamus, chitraka and sesame oil (YR)

Abbreviations Used

AH—Ashtanga hridaya.

BR—Bhaishajya ratnavali.

SS—Siddhayoga Sangraha

SY—Sahasrayoga

YR—Yogaratnakara

CD—Chakra Datta

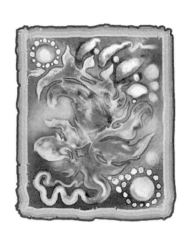

Bibliography

Bhavamishra. *Bhavaprakasha*. Prof. K.R. Srikantha Murthy translation. Varanasi, India: Krishnadas Academy, 2000.

Caraka. *Caraka Samhita*. R.K. Sharma and Bhagwan Dash translation. Varanasi, India: Chowkhamba Sanskrit Series Office, 1976.

Douillard, Dr. John. *Body, Mind and Sport*. New York, New York: Crown Trade Paperbacks , 1994.

Frawley, David. *The Astrology of the Seers*. Twin Lakes, Wis.: Lotus Press, 2000.

Frawley, David and Subhash Ranade. *Ayurveda: Nature's Medicine*. Twin Lakes, Wis.: Lotus Press, 2001.

Frawley, David. *Ayurvedic Healing*. Twin Lakes, Wis.: Lotus Press, 2000.

Frawley, David. *Yoga and Ayurveda*. Twin Lakes, Wis.: Lotus Press, 1999.

Frawley, David and Sandra Kozak. *Yoga for Your Type: An Ayurvedic Approach to Your Asana Practice*. Twin Lakes, Wis.: Lotus Press, 2001.

Frawley, David and Vasant Lad. *The Yoga of Herbs*. Twin Lakes, Wis.: Lotus Press, 1986.

Joshi, Dr. Sunil. *Ayurveda and Panchakarma*. Twin Lakes, Wis.: Lotus Press, 1997.

Lad, Dr. Vasant. *The Complete Book of Ayurvedic Home Remedies*. New York, New York: Harmony Books, 1998.

Lele, Dr. Avinash, Ranade and Qutab. *Pancha-Karma and Ayurvedic Massage*. Pune, India: International Academy of Ayurveda, 1998.

Miller, Light and Brian. *Ayurveda and Aromatherapy*. Twin Lakes, Wis.: Lotus Press, 1995.

Morningstar, Amadea. *The Ayurvedic Guide to Polarity Therapy*. Twin Lakes, Wis.: Lotus Press, 2001.

Pandey, Dr. Gyanendra. *Dravyaguna Vijnana* (three volumes). Varanasi, India: Krishnadas Academy, 1998.

Ranade, Dr. Subhash, Qutab and Deshpande. *Health and Disease in Ayurveda and Yoga.* Pune, India: Anmol Prakashan, 1998.

Ranade, Dr. Subhash, Qutab and Deshpande. *History and Philosophy of Ayurveda.* Pune, India: International Academy of Ayurveda, 1998.

Ros, Dr. Frank. *Ayurvedic Acupuncture.* Twin Lakes, Wis.: Lotus Press, 1993.

Selvara, John. *Varma Sutram 100* (Tamil Publication). Madras, India: I.I.T.S. Publication, 1984.

Simon, Dr. David. *Vital Energy.* New York, New York: John Wiley and Sons, 2000.

Smith, Atreya. *Prana: The Secret of Yogic Healing.* York Beach, Maine: Samuel Weiser, 1996.

Smith, Atreya. *Secrets of Ayurvedic Massage.* Twin Lakes, Wis.: Lotus Press, 1999.

Susruta. *Susruta Samhita.* P.V. Sharma translation. Varanasi, India: Chaukhambha Visvabharati, 1999.

Thatte, Dr. D.G. *Acupuncture, Marma and Other Asian Therapeutic Techniques.* Delhi, India: Chaukhamba Orientalia, 1976.

Tierra, Michael. *Planetary Herbology.* Twin Lakes, Wis.: Lotus Press, 1988.

Tirtha, Swami Sada Shiva. *The Ayurveda Encyclopedia.* Bayville, New York: Ayurvedic Holistic Center, 1998.

Van Howten, Donald. *Ayurveda and Life-Impressions Bodywork.* Twin Lakes, Wis.: Lotus Press, 1997.

Sanskrit Only

Ashtanga Hridaya of Vagbhatta.

Ashtanga Sangraha of Vagbhatta.

Gananath Sen. *Pratyakshasariram* (three volumes). Varanasi, India: Krishnadas Academy, 1998.

Vasishta Samhita. Lonavala, India; Kaivalya Dhama Sriman Madhva Yoga Mandira Samiti, 1984.

General Index

Index of Marmas

About the Authors & Resources

ABOUT THE AUTHORS

Dr. David Frawley (Pandit Vamadeva Shastri)

Dr. Frawley (Pandit Vamadeva Shastri) is regarded as one of the most important western exponents of Vedic knowledge in the world today. He has studied the Vedas, Puranas, Tantras and Yoga Shastras in the original Sanskrit and written extensively on their wisdom and their practices. He is the author of over twenty five books and numerous articles on diverse aspects of Vedic and Yogic knowledge, as well as several training programs on Ayurveda, Yoga and Vedic Astrology.

Dr. Frawley is a Pandit or traditional teacher of Vedic knowledge (Vedacharya), an Ayurvedacharya (traditional teacher of Ayurveda), Jyotish Brihaspati (professor of Vedic Astrology) and OMD (Oriental Medical Doctor). In India, where he has lectured and taught throughout the country, his Vedic work, including his translations from the Vedas, is highly regarded.

Dr. Frawley is the director of the American Institute of Vedic Studies and is also on the advisory boards for the National Association of Ayurvedic Medicine and the magazine *Yoga International*. He works closely with the California College of Ayurveda, the European Institute of Vedic Studies and the American College of Vedic Astrology.

Dr. Frawley is one the main western pioneers of Ayurvedic medicine, particularly relative to its interface with the greater system of Yoga. He presents detailed information for those who want to go deeply into these profound traditions. The aim of his work is to train serious students and practitioners, who can authentically represent the real teachings. He has a special connection with the teachings of Bhagavan Ramana Maharshi, which he has been involved with over the last thirty years.

American Institute of Vedic Studies

The American Institute of Vedic Studies is an educational center, directed by Dr. David Frawley, devoted to the greater systems of Vedic and Yogic knowledge. It teaches related aspects of Vedic Science including Ayurveda,

Vedic Astrology, Tantra, Yoga and Vedanta with a special reference to their background in the Vedas. It offers publications, courses and classes, including special tutorial programs for advanced students. The Institute is engaged in several research projects including:

- Ayurvedic Psychology and Yoga: The mental and spiritual aspects of Ayurveda and the Ayurvedic usage of Pranayama, Mantra and Meditation.
- Vedic Yoga: Restoring the ancient Vedic Yoga that perhaps is the foundation for the Yoga tradition, particularly the Vedic Agni or Fire Yoga.
- Translations and interpretations of the Vedas, particularly the Rig Veda.
- Vedic History: The history of India and of the world from a Vedic perspective, reflecting the latest archaeological work in India.
- The Soul and the Sacred Fire: Showing the ancient fire and enlightenment religion of all humanity.

The Institute, located in Santa Fe, New Mexico, has helped found various organizations including the European Institute of Vedic Studies, California College of Ayurveda, the American Council of Vedic Astrology, the World Association of Vedic Studies, the Vedic Friends Association, and the British Association of Vedic Astrology.

American Institute of Vedic Studies
PO Box 8357
Santa Fe, NM 87504-8357
Dr. David Frawley (Pandit Vamadeva Shastri), Director
Ph: 505-983-9385, Fax: 505-982-5807
Website: www.vedanet.com, Email: vedicinst@aol.com

American Institute of Vedic Studies
Ayurvedic Healing Correspondence Course

This comprehensive distance learning program covers all the main aspects of Ayurvedic theory, diagnosis and practice, with detailed information on herbal medicine and dietary therapy. It also goes in depth into Yoga philosophy and Ayurvedic psychology, outlining an integral mind-body medicine and its practical application. It contains the main material covered in two-year Ayurvedic programs for foreign students in India and more.

The course is designed for Health Care Professionals as well as for serious students to provide the foundation for becoming an Ayurvedic practitioner. It has been taken by doctors, chiropractors, nurses, acupuncturists, herbalists, massage therapists, yoga therapists and psychologists. However, there is no required medical background for those wishing to take the course and many non-professionals have completed it successfully. Topics include:

- Ayurvedic Anatomy and Physiology (Doshas, Dhatus, Malas, Srotas), Determination of Constitution, Diagnosis of Disease, the Disease Process, Samkhya and Yoga
- Diet and Nutrition, Ayurvedic Herbology, Pancha Karma, Aroma Therapy, Pranic Healing, Ayurvedic Psychology, Yoga and Ayurveda, Mantra and Meditation, and more.

The course is authored by Dr. David Frawley (Pandit Vamadeva Shastri), uses his books on Ayurveda and represents his approach to Ayurveda, adapting Ayurveda to the modern world without losing its spiritual integrity.

American Institute of Vedic Studies
Astrology of the Seers Correspondence Course

This comprehensive distance learning program explains Vedic Astrology in clear and modern terms, providing practical insights regarding how to adapt and use the system relative to our changing circumstances today. For those who have difficulty approaching the Vedic system, the course provides many keys for unlocking its language and its methodology for the western student.

The goal of the course is to provide the foundation to become a professional Vedic astrologer. Its orientation is two-fold: 1) to teach the language, approach and way of thinking of Vedic Astrology, and; 2) to teach the Astrology of Healing or Ayurvedic Astrology. Topics include:

- Planets, Signs, Houses, Aspects, Yogas, Nakshatras, Dashas, Divisional Charts, Ashtakavarga, Muhurta
- Ayurvedic (Medical) Astrology, Spiritual Astrology, Karma, Gem-therapy, Color-therapy, Mantras, Deities, and detailed Principles of Chart Analysis.

The course can be taken as part of a longer tutorial program of training in Vedic Astrology through the American Council of Vedic Astrology (ACVA), the largest Vedic Astrology organization outside of India. The course author, Dr. David Frawley, has been awarded the titles of Jyotish Kovid (proficiency in Vedic astrology) and Jyotish Brihaspati (Prof. of Vedic Astrology) through the Indian Council of Astrological Sciences (ICAS).

Prof. Subhash Ranade

Dr. Subhash Ranade is a leading academician and physician in the field of Ayurveda worldwide. He has written over sixty books on different aspects of Ayurveda, which have been published in Marathi, Hindi, Malayalam, Polish, Japanese, Italian and German. He has worked as Professor and Head of the Department of Ayurveda, Pune University and Principal of Ashtanga Ayurveda College in Pune, India.

At present Dr. Ranade is the Chairman of the International Academy of Ayurveda in Pune, which offers Ayurveda courses as well as Pancha Karma and Rejuvenative treatments for foreigners and Indians in Pune and Goa. He is also Chairman of the Ayurveda International Diffusing Association, Japan.

Professor Ranade has given many television interviews on Ayurveda, not only in India but in Poland, Italy and Germany as well. He has spoken at many international and national seminars on Ayurveda and Yoga. He has written numerous articles published in various magazines, newspapers in India and abroad and is also on the editorial board of several Ayurvedic journals.

He has had the honor of being visiting Professor to many Ayurvedic Institutes in the United States, the SEVA Academy in Munich, Germany, Ateneo Veda Vyasa, Savona, Italy and the Foundation for Health, Warsaw, Poland. He is in charge of the new Ayurveda courses that have been started at Barcelona, Spain and Graz, Austria.

His pioneering work in the field of CD-ROM'S like *Dhanvantari Ayurvedic Massage* and *Marma Therapy* have been whole-heartedly welcomed and highly appreciated. Since 1981, he has visited and conducted hundreds of Ayurveda courses for medical practitioners in Europe, USA, Canada and Japan.

Dr. Avinash Lele

Dr. Avinash Lele graduated from R. A. Podar Government Ayurvedic College in Mumbai with distinction in Ayurvedic surgery and did his post-graduate study from Tilak Ayurved College. He is an expert in Ayurvedic surgery, Pancha Karma and Rasayana (rejuvenation therapy), which he practices and teaches worldwide.

Dr. Lele has a broad professional experience having served as principal of Maharashtra Arogya Mandal's College of Ayurveda, Vice-President of Savitri Ayurved Pratishthan, Director of the International Academy of Ayurved, and professor of the Shalya Shalakya (surgery), Ashtang Ayurved College. He has been a post-graduate teacher and examiner since 1983. Dr. Lele has a vast clinical experience as Medical Director of Janaki Clinic and Panchakarma Health club, Chief Medical Consultant Atreya Rugnalaya and Research Center, and Director of Amrut Aushadhi which manufactures numerous Ayurvedic herbal products.

Dr. Lele is the author of several books on Ayurveda in both Marathi and English including Panchakarma and Ayurvedic Massage and Secrets of Marma. He has written many articles on different Ayurvedic subjects published in various journals in India and the West. He has organized various national scientific seminars and workshops on Ayurveda and conducted courses for foreign and Indian students with clinical training in Pancha Karma, Ayurvedic Massage, marma therapy, Ayurvedic acupressure and acupuncture and herbology.

Dr. Lele has been traveling and teaching Ayurveda worldwide since 1994 including Singapore, Japan, Hawaii, Bahamas, Italy, Switzerland, Netherlands, Austria, Germany and USA. He is a visiting professor and advisory board member for various institutions.

International Academy of Ayurveda

The International Academy of Ayurveda in Pune, India - whose chairman is Dr. Subhash Ranade and director is Dr. Avinash Lele-is one of the foremost institutions for training foreign students in India. It has complete facilities and programs for all levels of training from beginner to advanced, including special clinical instruction. It features a renowned faculty of Ayurvedic experts from throughout the world including Dr. Subhash Ranade, Dr. Avinash Lele, Dr. Abbas Qutab, Dr. Hans Rhyner, Dr. David Frawley and Mukunda Stiles. Pune itself is one of the most modern cities in India with a pleasant year round climate and easy airport access from Bombay (Mumbai), making it an ideal place in India to study.

The institute offers practical courses in Ayurveda, both basic and advanced. Special programs are available on the Fundamentals of Ayurveda, Pancha Karma, Ayurvedic Massage, Marma Therapy, Herbology and Clinical Studies. Programs are given July-August and November-January every year in batches of about ten students. Please register at least two months ahead of time to reserve your place.

The institute has its own line of a dozen important books on Ayurveda in English by Dr. Ranade, Dr. Lele, Dr. Frawley and others, as well as other educational materials (Ayurvedic CD-ROM) and herbal products, making it an important Ayurvedic resource center as well.

International Academy of Ayurveda
Nand Nandan, Atreya Rugnalaya, M.Y. Lele Chowk
Erandawana, Pune 411 004 India
Telefax: 91-11-212-378532/ 524427
Website: www.ayurveda-int.com

RESOURCES

Ayurveda Centers and Training

American Institute of Vedic Studies
Dr. David Frawley (Pandit Vamadeva
Shastri), Director
PO Box 8357
Santa Fe, NM 87504-8357
Ph: 505-983-9385
Fax: 505-982-5807
Email: vedicinst@aol.com
Website: www.vedanet.com

Aryavaidya Shala (Coimbatore)
136-137 Trichy Road
Coimbatore 641 045, T.N., India
Email: ayurveda@vsnl.com
Website: www.avpayurveda.com

**Australian College of
Ayurvedic Medicine**
Dr. Frank Ros, Director
PO Box 322
Ingle Farm S.A. 5098, Australia
Website: www.picknowl.com.au/
homepages/suchi-karma

Australian School of Ayurveda
Dr. Krishna Kumar, MD, FIIM
27 Blight Street
Ridleyton, South Australia 5008
Ph. 08-346-0631

Ayur-Veda AB
Box 78, 285 22 Markaryd
Esplanaden 2, Sweden
Ph: 0433-104 90
Fax: 0433-104 92
Email: info@ayur-veda.se

Ayurveda Academy
Dr. P.H. Kulkarni, President
36 Kothrud, Opp. Mhatoba Temple
Pune 411 029, India
Ph: 91-212-332130
Fax: 91-212-363132/ 343933.
Email: ayurveda.academy@jwbbs.com

Ayurveda for Radiant Health & Beauty
Ivy Amar
16 Espira Court
Santa Fe, NM 87505
Ph: 505-466-7662

Ayurvedic Holistic Center
Swami Sadashiva Tirtha, Director
82A Bayville Ave.
Bayville, NY 11709
Website: www.ayurvedahc.com

**Ayurvedic Institute and
Wellness Center**
Dr. Vasant Lad, Director
11311 Menaul, NE
Albuquerque, NM 87112
Ph: 505-291-9698
Website: www.ayurveda.com

**California Association of
Ayurvedic Medicine**
Website: www.ayurveda-caam.org

California College of Ayurveda
1117A East Main Street
Grass Valley, CA 95945
Ph: 530-274-9100
Email: info@ayurvedacollege.com
Website: www.ayurvedacollege.com
Two year state approved program in
Ayurveda

The Chopra Center
At La Costa Resort and Spa
Deepak Chopra and David Simon
7321 Estrella de Mar Road
Carlsbad, CA 93009
Ph: 888-424-6772
Website: www.chopra.com

John Douillard
Life Spa, Rejuvenation
through Ayurveda
3065 Center Green Dr.
Boulder, CO 80301
Ph: 303-442-1164
Website: www.LifeSpa.com

**East West College of Herbalism
Ayurvedic Program**
Hartswood, Marsh Green, Hartsfield
E. Sussex TN7 4ET, UK
Ph: 01342-822312
Fax: 01342-826346
Email: ewcolherb@aol.com

European Institute of Vedic Studies
Atreya Smith, Director
Editions Turiya
I.E.E.V sarl
B.P. 4
30170 Monoblet, France
Ph: (33) 466 85 04 11
Fax: (33) 466 85 0542
Website: www.atreya.com
Website: www.ayurvedicnutrition.com
Ayurvedic training in Europe

Ganesha Institute
Pratichi Mathur, President
4898 El Camino Real, Suite 203
Los Altos, CA 94022
Ph: 615-961-8316
Website: www.healingmission.com

Himalayan Institute
RR1, Box 400
Honesdale, PA 18431
Website: www.himalayaninstitute.org

Institute for Wholistic Education
Dept. MT
3425 Patzke Ln.
Racine WI 53405
Ph: 262-619-1798
Website: www.wholisticinstitute.org

International Academy of Ayurved
Dr. Avinash Lele
Nand Nandan, Atreya Rugnalaya
M.Y. Lele Chowk
Erandawana, Pune
411 004, India
Ph/Fax: 91-212-378532/524427
Email: avilele@hotmail.com

International Yoga Studies
Sandra Kozak, Director
692 Andrew Court
Benicia, CA 94510
Ph: 707-745-5224
Email: IYSUSA@aol.com.

Kaya Kalpa International
Dr. Raam Panday
111 Woodster Rd.
Satto, NY 10012

Kayakalpa
Sri Tatwamasi Dixit
22/2 Judge Jumbulingam Road
Off Radhakrishnan Salai, Mylapore
Chennai 600 004, India
Website: www.mypandit.com

Dr. Avinash Lele
Atreya Rugnalaya
Erandwana, Pune
India 411004
Tel/Fax: 91-20-5678532
Email: avilele@hotmail.com

Life Impressions Institute
Donald Van Howten, Director
613 Kathryn Street
Santa Fe, NM 87501
Ph: 505-988-2627

Light on Ayurveda: Journal of Health
Genevieve Ryder, Editor/Publisher
418-77 Quinaquisset Avenue
Mashpee, MA 02649
Ph: 508-477-4783
Website: www.loaj.com

Light Institute of Ayurveda
Dr.'s Bryan & Light Miller
PO Box 35284
Sarasota, FL 34242
Email: earthess@aol.com
Website: www.ayurvedichealings.com

Lotus Ayurvedic Center
4145 Clares St., Suite D
Capitola, CA 95010
Ph: 408-479-1667
Website: www.lotusayurveda.com

Lotus Press
Dept. MT
PO Box 325
Twin Lakes, WI 53181
Ph: 262-889-8561
Fax: 262-889-2461
Email: lotuspress@lotuspress.com
Website: www.lotuspress.com
Publisher of books on Ayurveda, Reiki,
aromatherapy, energetic healing, herbal-
ism, alternative health and U.S. editions
of Sri Aurobindo's writings.

National Association of Ayurvedic Medicine
Website: www.ayurvedic-association.org

National Institute of Ayurvedic Medicine
584 Milltown Road
Brewster, NY 10509
Ph: 845-278-8700
Email: niam@niam.com
Website: www.niam.com

Dr. Subhash Ranade
Rajbharati, 367 Sahakar Nagar 1
Pune 411 009, India
Email: sbranade@hotmail.com

Rocky Mountain Institute of Yoga and Ayurveda
PO Box 1091
Boulder, CO 80306
Ph: 303-499-2910
Email: rmiya@earthnet.net
Website: www.rmiya.org

Sanskrit Sounds - Nicolai Bachman
PO Box 4352
Santa Fe, NM 87502
Email: shabda@earthlink.net
Website: www.SanskritSounds.com

Texas Yoga & Ayurveda Institute
Dr. Rob Francis, director
4008 Vista Rd., Bldg. B, Suite 201
Pasadena, Texas 77504
Ph: 713-941-9642
Website: www.texasyoga.net

Vinayak Ayurveda Center
2509 Virginia NE, Suite D
Albuquerque, NM 87110
Ph: 505-296-6522
Website: www.vinayakayurveda.com

Vedic Cultural Fellowship
Howard Beckman, Director
HC 70, Box 620
Pecos, NM 87552
Ph: 505-757-6194
Website: www.vedicworld.org

Wise Earth School of Ayurveda
Bri. Maya Tiwari

90 Davis Creek Road
Candler, NC 28715
Ph: 828-258-9999
Website: www.wisearth.org

Ayurvedic Herbal Suppliers

Auroma International
Dept. MT
PO Box 1008
Silver Lake, WI 53170
Ph: 262-889-8569
Fax: 262-889-2461
Email: auroma@lotuspress.com
Website: www.auromaintl.com
Importer and master distributor of Auroshikha Incense, Chandrika Ayurvedic Soap and Herbal Vedic Ayurvedic products.

Ayur Herbal Corporation
PO Box 6390
Santa Fe, NM 87502
Ph: 262-889-8569
Website: www.herbalvedic.com
Manufacturer of Herbal Vedic Ayurvedic products.

Ayush Herbs, Inc.
10025 N.E. 4th Street
Bellevue, WA 98004
Ph: 800-925-1371

Banyan Trading Company
PO Box 13002
Albuquerque, NM 87192
Ph: 505-244-1880; 800-953-6424
Website: www.banyantrading.com
Traditional Ayurvedic Herbs - Wholesale

Bazaar of India Imports
1810 University Avenue
Berkeley, CA 94703
Ph: 800-261-7662; 510-548-4110
Website: www.bazaarofindia.com

Bio Veda
215 North Route 303
Congers, NY 10920-1726
Ph: 800-292-6002

Earth Essentials Florida
Dr.'s Bryan and Light Miller
4067 Shell Road
Sarasota, FL 34242
Ph: 941-316-0920
Email: earthess@aol.com
Website: www.ayurvedichealings.com

Frontier Herbs
PO Box 229
Norway, IA 52318
Ph: 800-669-3275

HerbalVedic Products
PO Box 6390
Santa Fe, NM 87502
Website: www.herbalvedic.com

Internatural
Dept. MT
PO Box 489
Twin Lakes, WI 53181
800-643-4221 (toll free order line)
262-889-8581 (office phone)
262-889-8591 (fax)
Email: internatural@lotuspress.com
Website: www.internatural.com
Retail mail order and Internet re-seller of Ayurvedic products, essential oils, herbs, spices, supplements, herbal remedies, incense, books, yoga mats, supplies and videos.

Lotus Brands, Inc.
Dept. MT
PO Box 325
Twin Lakes, WI 53181
Ph: 262-889-8561
Fax: 262-889-2461
Email: lotusbrands@lotuspress.com
Website: www.lotusbrands.com

Lotus Herbs
1505 42nd Ave., Suite 19
Capitola, CA 95010
Ph: 408-479-1667
Website: www.lotusayurveda.com

Lotus Light Enterprises
Dept. MT
PO Box 1008
Silver Lake, WI 53170

800-548-3824 (toll free order line)
262-889-8501 (office phone)
262-889-8591 (fax)
Email: lotuslight@lotuspress.com
Website: www.lotuslight.com
Wholesale distributor of Ayurvedic products, essential oils, herbs, spices, supplements, herbal remedies, incense, books and other supplies. Must supply resale certificate number or practitioner license to obtain catalog of more than 10,000 items.

Maharishi Ayurveda Products International
417 Bolton Road
PO Box 541
Lancaster, MA 01523
Info: 800-843-8332 Ext. 903
Order: 800-255-8332 Ext. 903

Om Organics
3245 Prairie Avenue, Suite A
Boulder, CO 80301
Ph: 888-550-VEDA
Website: www.omorganics.com

Organic India
Affiliate of Om Organics
Indira Nager, Lucknow,
Uttar Pradesh, 226016, India
Website: www.organicindia.com

Planetary Formulations
PO Box 533
Soquel, CA 95073
Website: www.planetherbs.com
Formulas by Dr. Michael Tierra

Tri Health
Jeff Lindner, Director
Kauai, Hawaii
Ph: 800-455-0770
Email: oilbath@aloha.net
Website: www.oilbath.com
Ayurvedic herbs and formulas from the Kerala Ayurvedic Pharmacy

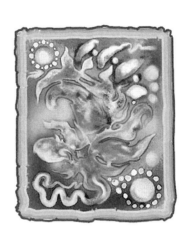

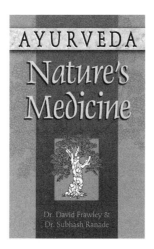

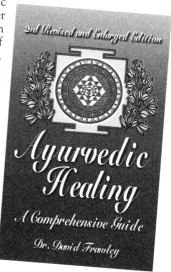

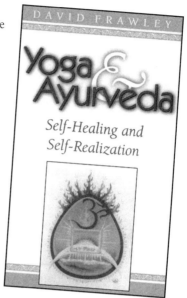

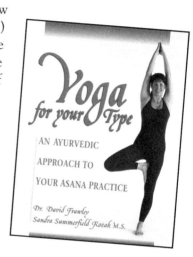